PSB
Practical Nursing Exam

SECRETS

Study Guide
Your Key to Exam Success

PSB Test Review for the
Psychological Services Bureau, Inc (PSB)
Practical Nursing Exam

Dear Future Exam Success Story:

First of all, **THANK YOU** for purchasing Mometrix study materials!

Second, congratulations! You are one of the few determined test-takers who are committed to doing whatever it takes to excel on your exam. **You have come to the right place.** We developed these study materials with one goal in mind: to deliver you the information you need in a format that's concise and easy to use.

In addition to optimizing your guide for the content of the test, we've outlined our recommended steps for breaking down the preparation process into small, attainable goals so you can make sure you stay on track.

We've also analyzed the entire test-taking process, identifying the most common pitfalls and showing how you can overcome them and be ready for any curveball the test throws you.

Standardized testing is one of the biggest obstacles on your road to success, which only increases the importance of doing well in the high-pressure, high-stakes environment of test day. Your results on this test could have a significant impact on your future, and this guide provides the information and practical advice to help you achieve your full potential on test day.

Your success is our success

We would love to hear from you! If you would like to share the story of your exam success or if you have any questions or comments in regard to our products, please contact us at **800-673-8175** or **support@mometrix.com**.

Thanks again for your business and we wish you continued success!

Sincerely,
The Mometrix Test Preparation Team

Need more help? Check out our flashcards at: http://MometrixFlashcards.com/PSB

TABLE OF CONTENTS

Introduction

Thank you for purchasing this resource! You have made the choice to prepare yourself for a test that could have a huge impact on your future, and this guide is designed to help you be fully ready for test day. Obviously, it's important to have a solid understanding of the test material, but you also need to be prepared for the unique environment and stressors of the test, so that you can perform to the best of your abilities.

For this purpose, the first section that appears in this guide is the **Secret Keys**. We've devoted countless hours to meticulously researching what works and what doesn't, and we've boiled down our findings to the five most impactful steps you can take to improve your performance on the test. We start at the beginning with study planning and move through the preparation process, all the way to the testing strategies that will help you get the most out of what you know when you're finally sitting in front of the test.

We recommend that you start preparing for your test as far in advance as possible. However, if you've bought this guide as a last-minute study resource and only have a few days before your test, we recommend that you skip over the first two Secret Keys since they address a long-term study plan.

If you struggle with **test anxiety**, we strongly encourage you to check out our recommendations for how you can overcome it. Test anxiety is a formidable foe, but it can be beaten, and we want to make sure you have the tools you need to defeat it.

Secret Key #1 – Plan Big, Study Small

There's a lot riding on your performance. If you want to ace this test, you're going to need to keep your skills sharp and the material fresh in your mind. You need a plan that lets you review everything you need to know while still fitting in your schedule. We'll break this strategy down into three categories.

Information Organization

Start with the information you already have: the official test outline. From this, you can make a complete list of all the concepts you need to cover before the test. Organize these concepts into groups that can be studied together, and create a list of any related vocabulary you need to learn so you can brush up on any difficult terms. You'll want to keep this vocabulary list handy once you actually start studying since you may need to add to it along the way.

Time Management

Once you have your set of study concepts, decide how to spread them out over the time you have left before the test. Break your study plan into small, clear goals so you have a manageable task for each day and know exactly what you're doing. Then just focus on one small step at a time. When you manage your time this way, you don't need to spend hours at a time studying. Studying a small block of content for a short period each day helps you retain information better and avoid stressing over how much you have left to do. You can relax knowing that you have a plan to cover everything in time. In order for this strategy to be effective though, you have to start studying early and stick to your schedule. Avoid the exhaustion and futility that comes from last-minute cramming!

Study Environment

The environment you study in has a big impact on your learning. Studying in a coffee shop, while probably more enjoyable, is not likely to be as fruitful as studying in a quiet room. It's important to keep distractions to a minimum. You're only planning to study for a short block of time, so make the most of it. Don't pause to check your phone or get up to find a snack. It's also important to **avoid multitasking**. Research has consistently shown that multitasking will make your studying dramatically less effective. Your study area should also be comfortable and well-lit so you don't have the distraction of straining your eyes or sitting on an uncomfortable chair.

The time of day you study is also important. You want to be rested and alert. Don't wait until just before bedtime. Study when you'll be most likely to comprehend and remember. Even better, if you know what time of day your test will be, set that time aside for study. That way your brain will be used to working on that subject at that specific time and you'll have a better chance of recalling information.

Finally, it can be helpful to team up with others who are studying for the same test. Your actual studying should be done in as isolated an environment as possible, but the work of organizing the information and setting up the study plan can be divided up. In between study sessions, you can discuss with your teammates the concepts that you're all studying and quiz each other on the details. Just be sure that your teammates are as serious about the test as you are. If you find that your study time is being replaced with social time, you might need to find a new team.

Secret Key #2 – Make Your Studying Count

You're devoting a lot of time and effort to preparing for this test, so you want to be absolutely certain it will pay off. This means doing more than just reading the content and hoping you can remember it on test day. It's important to make every minute of study count. There are two main areas you can focus on to make your studying count:

Retention

It doesn't matter how much time you study if you can't remember the material. You need to make sure you are retaining the concepts. To check your retention of the information you're learning, try recalling it at later times with minimal prompting. Try carrying around flashcards and glance at one or two from time to time or ask a friend who's also studying for the test to quiz you.

To enhance your retention, look for ways to put the information into practice so that you can apply it rather than simply recalling it. If you're using the information in practical ways, it will be much easier to remember. Similarly, it helps to solidify a concept in your mind if you're not only reading it to yourself but also explaining it to someone else. Ask a friend to let you teach them about a concept you're a little shaky on (or speak aloud to an imaginary audience if necessary). As you try to summarize, define, give examples, and answer your friend's questions, you'll understand the concepts better and they will stay with you longer. Finally, step back for a big picture view and ask yourself how each piece of information fits with the whole subject. When you link the different concepts together and see them working together as a whole, it's easier to remember the individual components.

Finally, practice showing your work on any multi-step problems, even if you're just studying. Writing out each step you take to solve a problem will help solidify the process in your mind, and you'll be more likely to remember it during the test.

Modality

Modality simply refers to the means or method by which you study. Choosing a study modality that fits your own individual learning style is crucial. No two people learn best in exactly the same way, so it's important to know your strengths and use them to your advantage.

For example, if you learn best by visualization, focus on visualizing a concept in your mind and draw an image or a diagram. Try color-coding your notes, illustrating them, or creating symbols that will trigger your mind to recall a learned concept. If you learn best by hearing or discussing information, find a study partner who learns the same way or read aloud to yourself. Think about how to put the information in your own words. Imagine that you are giving a lecture on the topic and record yourself so you can listen to it later.

For any learning style, flashcards can be helpful. Organize the information so you can take advantage of spare moments to review. Underline key words or phrases. Use different colors for different categories. Mnemonic devices (such as creating a short list in which every item starts with the same letter) can also help with retention. Find what works best for you and use it to store the information in your mind most effectively and easily.

Secret Key #3 – Practice the Right Way

Your success on test day depends not only on how many hours you put into preparing, but also on whether you prepared the right way. It's good to check along the way to see if your studying is paying off. One of the most effective ways to do this is by taking practice tests to evaluate your progress. Practice tests are useful because they show exactly where you need to improve. Every time you take a practice test, pay special attention to these three groups of questions:

- The questions you got wrong
- The questions you had to guess on, even if you guessed right
- The questions you found difficult or slow to work through

This will show you exactly what your weak areas are, and where you need to devote more study time. Ask yourself why each of these questions gave you trouble. Was it because you didn't understand the material? Was it because you didn't remember the vocabulary? Do you need more repetitions on this type of question to build speed and confidence? Dig into those questions and figure out how you can strengthen your weak areas as you go back to review the material.

Additionally, many practice tests have a section explaining the answer choices. It can be tempting to read the explanation and think that you now have a good understanding of the concept. However, an explanation likely only covers part of the question's broader context. Even if the explanation makes sense, **go back and investigate** every concept related to the question until you're positive you have a thorough understanding.

As you go along, keep in mind that the practice test is just that: practice. Memorizing these questions and answers will not be very helpful on the actual test because it is unlikely to have any of the same exact questions. If you only know the right answers to the sample questions, you won't be prepared for the real thing. **Study the concepts** until you understand them fully, and then you'll be able to answer any question that shows up on the test.

It's important to wait on the practice tests until you're ready. If you take a test on your first day of study, you may be overwhelmed by the amount of material covered and how much you need to learn. Work up to it gradually.

On test day, you'll need to be prepared for answering questions, managing your time, and using the test-taking strategies you've learned. It's a lot to balance, like a mental marathon that will have a big impact on your future. Like training for a marathon, you'll need to start slowly and work your way up. When test day arrives, you'll be ready.

Start with the strategies you've read in the first two Secret Keys—plan your course and study in the way that works best for you. If you have time, consider using multiple study resources to get different approaches to the same concepts. It can be helpful to see difficult concepts from more than one angle. Then find a good source for practice tests. Many times, the test website will suggest potential study resources or provide sample tests.

Practice Test Strategy

When you're ready to start taking practice tests, follow this strategy:

Untimed and Open-Book Practice

Take the first test with no time constraints and with your notes and study guide handy. Take your time and focus on applying the strategies you've learned.

Timed and Open-Book Practice

Take the second practice test open-book as well, but set a timer and practice pacing yourself to finish in time.

Timed and Closed-Book Practice

Take any other practice tests as if it were test day. Set a timer and put away your study materials. Sit at a table or desk in a quiet room, imagine yourself at the testing center, and answer questions as quickly and accurately as possible.

Keep repeating timed and closed-book tests on a regular basis until you run out of practice tests or it's time for the actual test. Your mind will be ready for the schedule and stress of test day, and you'll be able to focus on recalling the material you've learned.

Secret Key #4 – Pace Yourself

Once you're fully prepared for the material on the test, your biggest challenge on test day will be managing your time. Just knowing that the clock is ticking can make you panic even if you have plenty of time left. Work on pacing yourself so you can build confidence against the time constraints of the exam. Pacing is a difficult skill to master, especially in a high-pressure environment, so **practice is vital**.

Set time expectations for your pace based on how much time is available. For example, if a section has 60 questions and the time limit is 30 minutes, you know you have to average 30 seconds or less per question in order to answer them all. Although 30 seconds is the hard limit, set 25 seconds per question as your goal, so you reserve extra time to spend on harder questions. When you budget extra time for the harder questions, you no longer have any reason to stress when those questions take longer to answer.

Don't let this time expectation distract you from working through the test at a calm, steady pace, but keep it in mind so you don't spend too much time on any one question. Recognize that taking extra time on one question you don't understand may keep you from answering two that you do understand later in the test. If your time limit for a question is up and you're still not sure of the answer, mark it and move on, and come back to it later if the time and the test format allow. If the testing format doesn't allow you to return to earlier questions, just make an educated guess; then put it out of your mind and move on.

On the easier questions, be careful not to rush. It may seem wise to hurry through them so you have more time for the challenging ones, but it's not worth missing one if you know the concept and just didn't take the time to read the question fully. Work efficiently but make sure you understand the question and have looked at all of the answer choices, since more than one may seem right at first.

Even if you're paying attention to the time, you may find yourself a little behind at some point. You should speed up to get back on track, but do so wisely. Don't panic; just take a few seconds less on each question until you're caught up. Don't guess without thinking, but do look through the answer choices and eliminate any you know are wrong. If you can get down to two choices, it is often worthwhile to guess from those. Once you've chosen an answer, move on and don't dwell on any that you skipped or had to hurry through. If a question was taking too long, chances are it was one of the harder ones, so you weren't as likely to get it right anyway.

On the other hand, if you find yourself getting ahead of schedule, it may be beneficial to slow down a little. The more quickly you work, the more likely you are to make a careless mistake that will affect your score. You've budgeted time for each question, so don't be afraid to spend that time. Practice an efficient but careful pace to get the most out of the time you have.

Secret Key #5 – Have a Plan for Guessing

When you're taking the test, you may find yourself stuck on a question. Some of the answer choices seem better than others, but you don't see the one answer choice that is obviously correct. What do you do?

The scenario described above is very common, yet most test takers have not effectively prepared for it. Developing and practicing a plan for guessing may be one of the single most effective uses of your time as you get ready for the exam.

In developing your plan for guessing, there are three questions to address:

- When should you start the guessing process?
- How should you narrow down the choices?
- Which answer should you choose?

When to Start the Guessing Process

Unless your plan for guessing is to select C every time (which, despite its merits, is not what we recommend), you need to leave yourself enough time to apply your answer elimination strategies. Since you have a limited amount of time for each question, that means that if you're going to give yourself the best shot at guessing correctly, you have to decide quickly whether or not you will guess.

Of course, the best-case scenario is that you don't have to guess at all, so first, see if you can answer the question based on your knowledge of the subject and basic reasoning skills. Focus on the key words in the question and try to jog your memory of related topics. Give yourself a chance to bring the knowledge to mind, but once you realize that you don't have (or you can't access) the knowledge you need to answer the question, it's time to start the guessing process.

It's almost always better to start the guessing process too early than too late. It only takes a few seconds to remember something and answer the question from knowledge. Carefully eliminating wrong answer choices takes longer. Plus, going through the process of eliminating answer choices can actually help jog your memory.

Summary: Start the guessing process as soon as you decide that you can't answer the question based on your knowledge.

How to Narrow Down the Choices

The next chapter in this book (**Test-Taking Strategies**) includes a wide range of strategies for how to approach questions and how to look for answer choices to eliminate. You will definitely want to read those carefully, practice them, and figure out which ones work best for you. Here though, we're going to address a mindset rather than a particular strategy.

Your chances of guessing an answer correctly depend on how many options you are choosing from.

How many choices you have	How likely you are to guess correctly
5	20%
4	25%
3	33%
2	50%
1	100%

You can see from this chart just how valuable it is to be able to eliminate incorrect answers and make an educated guess, but there are two things that many test takers do that cause them to miss out on the benefits of guessing:

- Accidentally eliminating the correct answer
- Selecting an answer based on an impression

We'll look at the first one here, and the second one in the next section.

To avoid accidentally eliminating the correct answer, we recommend a thought exercise called **the $5 challenge**. In this challenge, you only eliminate an answer choice from contention if you are willing to bet $5 on it being wrong. Why $5? Five dollars is a small but not insignificant amount of money. It's an amount you could afford to lose but wouldn't want to throw away. And while losing $5 once might not hurt too much, doing it twenty times will set you back $100. In the same way, each small decision you make—eliminating a choice here, guessing on a question there—won't by itself impact your score very much, but when you put them all together, they can make a big difference. By holding each answer choice elimination decision to a higher standard, you can reduce the risk of accidentally eliminating the correct answer.

The $5 challenge can also be applied in a positive sense: If you are willing to bet $5 that an answer choice *is* correct, go ahead and mark it as correct.

Summary: Only eliminate an answer choice if you are willing to bet $5 that it is wrong.

Which Answer to Choose

You're taking the test. You've run into a hard question and decided you'll have to guess. You've eliminated all the answer choices you're willing to bet $5 on. Now you have to pick an answer. Why do we even need to talk about this? Why can't you just pick whichever one you feel like when the time comes?

The answer to these questions is that if you don't come into the test with a plan, you'll rely on your impression to select an answer choice, and if you do that, you risk falling into a trap. The test writers know that everyone who takes their test will be guessing on some of the questions, so they intentionally write wrong answer choices to seem plausible. You still have to pick an answer though, and if the wrong answer choices are designed to look right, how can you ever be sure that you're not falling for their trap? The best solution we've found to this dilemma is to take the decision out of your hands entirely. Here is the process we recommend:

Once you've eliminated any choices that you are confident (willing to bet $5) are wrong, select the first remaining choice as your answer.

Whether you choose to select the first remaining choice, the second, or the last, the important thing is that you use some preselected standard. Using this approach guarantees that you will not be enticed into selecting an answer choice that looks right, because you are not basing your decision on how the answer choices look.

This is not meant to make you question your knowledge. Instead, it is to help you recognize the difference between your knowledge and your impressions. There's a huge difference between thinking an answer is right because of what you know, and thinking an answer is right because it looks or sounds like it should be right.

Summary: To ensure that your selection is appropriately random, make a predetermined selection from among all answer choices you have not eliminated.

Test-Taking Strategies

This section contains a list of test-taking strategies that you may find helpful as you work through the test. By taking what you know and applying logical thought, you can maximize your chances of answering any question correctly!

It is very important to realize that every question is different and every person is different: no single strategy will work on every question, and no single strategy will work for every person. That's why we've included all of them here, so you can try them out and determine which ones work best for different types of questions and which ones work best for you.

Question Strategies

Read Carefully

Read the question and answer choices carefully. Don't miss the question because you misread the terms. You have plenty of time to read each question thoroughly and make sure you understand what is being asked. Yet a happy medium must be attained, so don't waste too much time. You must read carefully, but efficiently.

Contextual Clues

Look for contextual clues. If the question includes a word you are not familiar with, look at the immediate context for some indication of what the word might mean. Contextual clues can often give you all the information you need to decipher the meaning of an unfamiliar word. Even if you can't determine the meaning, you may be able to narrow down the possibilities enough to make a solid guess at the answer to the question.

Prefixes

If you're having trouble with a word in the question or answer choices, try dissecting it. Take advantage of every clue that the word might include. Prefixes and suffixes can be a huge help. Usually they allow you to determine a basic meaning. Pre- means before, post- means after, pro - is positive, de- is negative. From prefixes and suffixes, you can get an idea of the general meaning of the word and try to put it into context.

Hedge Words

Watch out for critical hedge words, such as *likely, may, can, sometimes, often, almost, mostly, usually, generally, rarely,* and *sometimes.* Question writers insert these hedge phrases to cover every possibility. Often an answer choice will be wrong simply because it leaves no room for exception. Be on guard for answer choices that have definitive words such as *exactly* and *always.*

Switchback Words

Stay alert for *switchbacks.* These are the words and phrases frequently used to alert you to shifts in thought. The most common switchback words are *but, although,* and *however.* Others include *nevertheless, on the other hand, even though, while, in spite of, despite, regardless of.* Switchback words are important to catch because they can change the direction of the question or an answer choice.

Face Value

When in doubt, use common sense. Accept the situation in the problem at face value. Don't read too much into it. These problems will not require you to make wild assumptions. If you have to go beyond creativity and warp time or space in order to have an answer choice fit the question, then you should move on and consider the other answer choices. These are normal problems rooted in reality. The applicable relationship or explanation may not be readily apparent, but it is there for you to figure out. Use your common sense to interpret anything that isn't clear.

Answer Choice Strategies

Answer Selection

The most thorough way to pick an answer choice is to identify and eliminate wrong answers until only one is left, then confirm it is the correct answer. Sometimes an answer choice may immediately seem right, but be careful. The test writers will usually put more than one reasonable answer choice on each question, so take a second to read all of them and make sure that the other choices are not equally obvious. As long as you have time left, it is better to read every answer choice than to pick the first one that looks right without checking the others.

Answer Choice Families

An answer choice family consists of two (in rare cases, three) answer choices that are very similar in construction and cannot all be true at the same time. If you see two answer choices that are direct opposites or parallels, one of them is usually the correct answer. For instance, if one answer choice says that quantity x increases and another either says that quantity x decreases (opposite) or says that quantity y increases (parallel), then those answer choices would fall into the same family. An answer choice that doesn't match the construction of the answer choice family is more likely to be incorrect. Most questions will not have answer choice families, but when they do appear, you should be prepared to recognize them.

Eliminate Answers

Eliminate answer choices as soon as you realize they are wrong, but make sure you consider all possibilities. If you are eliminating answer choices and realize that the last one you are left with is also wrong, don't panic. Start over and consider each choice again. There may be something you missed the first time that you will realize on the second pass.

Avoid Fact Traps

Don't be distracted by an answer choice that is factually true but doesn't answer the question. You are looking for the choice that answers the question. Stay focused on what the question is asking for so you don't accidentally pick an answer that is true but incorrect. Always go back to the question and make sure the answer choice you've selected actually answers the question and is not merely a true statement.

Extreme Statements

In general, you should avoid answers that put forth extreme actions as standard practice or proclaim controversial ideas as established fact. An answer choice that states the "process should be used in certain situations, if..." is much more likely to be correct than one that states the "process should be discontinued completely." The first is a calm rational statement and doesn't even make a definitive, uncompromising stance, using a hedge word *if* to provide wiggle room, whereas the second choice is a radical idea and far more extreme.

Benchmark

As you read through the answer choices and you come across one that seems to answer the question well, mentally select that answer choice. This is not your final answer, but it's the one that will help you evaluate the other answer choices. The one that you selected is your benchmark or standard for judging each of the other answer choices. Every other answer choice must be compared to your benchmark. That choice is correct until proven otherwise by another answer choice beating it. If you find a better answer, then that one becomes your new benchmark. Once you've decided that no other choice answers the question as well as your benchmark, you have your final answer.

Predict the Answer

Before you even start looking at the answer choices, it is often best to try to predict the answer. When you come up with the answer on your own, it is easier to avoid distractions and traps because you will know exactly what to look for. The right answer choice is unlikely to be word-for-word what you came up with, but it should be a close match. Even if you are confident that you have the right answer, you should still take the time to read each option before moving on.

General Strategies

Tough Questions

If you are stumped on a problem or it appears too hard or too difficult, don't waste time. Move on! Remember though, if you can quickly check for obviously incorrect answer choices, your chances of guessing correctly are greatly improved. Before you completely give up, at least try to knock out a couple of possible answers. Eliminate what you can and then guess at the remaining answer choices before moving on.

Check Your Work

Since you will probably not know every term listed and the answer to every question, it is important that you get credit for the ones that you do know. Don't miss any questions through careless mistakes. If at all possible, try to take a second to look back over your answer selection and make sure you've selected the correct answer choice and haven't made a costly careless mistake (such as marking an answer choice that you didn't mean to mark). This quick double check should more than pay for itself in caught mistakes for the time it costs.

Pace Yourself

It's easy to be overwhelmed when you're looking at a page full of questions; your mind is confused and full of random thoughts, and the clock is ticking down faster than you would like. Calm down and maintain the pace that you have set for yourself. Especially as you get down to the last few minutes of the test, don't let the small numbers on the clock make you panic. As long as you are on track by monitoring your pace, you are guaranteed to have time for each question.

Don't Rush

It is very easy to make errors when you are in a hurry. Maintaining a fast pace in answering questions is pointless if it makes you miss questions that you would have gotten right otherwise. Test writers like to include distracting information and wrong answers that seem right. Taking a little extra time to avoid careless mistakes can make all the difference in your test score. Find a pace that allows you to be confident in the answers that you select.

Keep Moving

Panicking will not help you pass the test, so do your best to stay calm and keep moving. Taking deep breaths and going through the answer elimination steps you practiced can help to break through a stress barrier and keep your pace.

Final Notes

The combination of a solid foundation of content knowledge and the confidence that comes from practicing your plan for applying that knowledge is the key to maximizing your performance on test day. As your foundation of content knowledge is built up and strengthened, you'll find that the strategies included in this chapter become more and more effective in helping you quickly sift through the distractions and traps of the test to isolate the correct answer.

Now it's time to move on to the test content chapters of this book, but be sure to keep your goal in mind. As you read, think about how you will be able to apply this information on the test. If you've already seen sample questions for the test and you have an idea of the question format and style, try to come up with questions of your own that you can answer based on what you're reading. This will give you valuable practice applying your knowledge in the same ways you can expect to on test day.

Good luck and good studying!

Part I- Vocabulary Review

The Vocabulary test on the exam consists of 30 questions about Word Knowledge.

Word Knowledge

Nearly and Perfect Synonyms

You must determine which of four provided choices has the best similar definition as a certain word. Nearly similar may often be more correct, because the goal is to test your understanding of the nuances, or little differences, between words. A perfect match may not exist, so don't be concerned if your answer choice is not a complete synonym. Focus upon edging closer to the word. Eliminate the words that you know aren't correct first. Then narrow your search. Cross out the words that are the least similar to the main word until you are left with the one that is the most similar.

Prefixes

Take advantage of every clue that the word might include. Prefixes and suffixes can be a huge help. Usually they allow you to determine a basic meaning. Pre- means before, post- means after, pro – is positive, de- is negative. From these prefixes and suffixes, you can get an idea of the general meaning of the word and look for its opposite. Beware though of any traps. Just because con is the opposite of pro, doesn't necessarily mean congress is the opposite of progress! A list of the most common prefixes and suffixes is included in a special report at the end.

> **Review Video: Prefixes**
> Visit mometrix.com/academy and enter code: 361382

Positive vs. Negative

Many words can be easily determined to be a positive word or a negative word. Words such as despicable, gruesome, and bleak are all negative. Words such as ecstatic, praiseworthy, and magnificent are all positive. You will be surprised at how many words can be considered as either positive or negative. Once that is determined, you can quickly eliminate any other words with an opposite meaning and focus on those that have the other characteristic, whether positive or negative.

Word Strength

Part of the challenge is determining the most nearly similar word. This is particularly true when two words seem to be similar. When analyzing a word, determine how strong it is. For example, stupendous and good are both positive words.

However, stupendous is a much stronger positive adjective than good. Also, towering or gigantic are stronger words than tall or large. Search for an answer choice that is similar and also has the same strength. If the main word is weak, look for similar words that are also weak. If the main word is strong, look for similar words that are also strong.

Type and Topic

Another key is what type of word is the main word. If the main word is an adjective describing height, then look for the answer to be an adjective describing height as well. Match both the type and topic of the main word. The type refers the parts of speech, whether the word is an adjective, adverb, or verb. The topic refers to what the definition of the word includes, such as sizes or fashion styles.

> **Review Video: Word Types**
> Visit mometrix.com/academy and enter code: 964551

Form a Sentence

Many words seem more natural in a sentence. *Specious* reasoning, *irresistible* force, and *uncanny* resemblance are just a few of the word combinations that usually go together. When faced with an uncommon word that you barely understand, try to put the word in a sentence that makes sense. It will help you to understand the word's meaning and make it easier to determine its opposite. Once you have a good descriptive sentence that utilizes the main word properly, plug in the answer choices and see if the sentence still has the same meaning with each answer choice. The answer choice that maintains the meaning of the sentence is correct!

Use Replacements

Using a sentence is a great help because it puts the word into a proper perspective. Since the exam actually gives you a sentence, sometimes you don't always have to create your own (though in many cases the sentence won't be helpful). Read the provided sentence, picking out the main word. Then read the sentence again and again, each time replacing the main word with one of the answer choices. The correct answer should "sound" right and fit.

Example: The desert landscape was desolate. Desolate means:

1. cheerful
2. creepy
3. excited
4. forlorn

After reading the example sentence, begin replacing "desolate" with each of the answer choices. Does "the desert landscape was cheerful, creepy, excited, or forlorn" sound right? Deserts are typically hot, empty, and rugged environments, probably not cheerful, or excited. While creepy might sound right, that word would certainly be more appropriate for a haunted house. But "the desert landscape was forlorn" has a certain ring to it and would be correct.

Eliminate Similar Choices

If you don't know the word, don't worry. Look at the answer choices and just use them. Remember that three of the answer choices will always be wrong. If you can find a common relationship between any three answer choices, then you know they are wrong. Find the answer choice that does not have a common relationship to the other answer choices and it will be the correct answer.

Example: Laconic most nearly means

1. wordy
2. talkative
3. expressive
4. quiet

In this example, the first three choices are all similar. Even if you don't know that laconic means the same as quiet, you know that "quiet" must be correct, because the other three choices were all virtually the same. They were all the same, so they must all be wrong. The one that is different must be correct. So, don't worry if you don't know a word. Focus on the answer choices that you do understand and see if you can identify similarities. Even identifying two words that are similar will allow you to eliminate those two answer choices. Because they are similar, they are either both right or both wrong, and since they can't both be right, they must both be wrong.

Example: He worked slowly, moving the leather back and forth until it was ____.

1. rough
2. hard
3. stiff
4. pliable

In this example the first three choices are all similar and synonyms. Even without knowing what pliable means, it has to be correct, because you know the other three answer choices mean the same thing.

Adjectives Give it Away

Words mean things and are added to the sentence for a reason. Adjectives in particular may be the clue to determining which answer choice is correct.

Example: The brilliant scientist made several discoveries that were

1. dull
2. dazzling

Look at the adjectives first to help determine what makes sense. A "brilliant" or smart scientist would make dazzling, rather than dull discoveries. Without that simple adjective, no answer choice is clear.

Use Logic

Ask yourself questions about each answer choice to see if they are logical.

Example: In the distance, the deep pounding resonance of the drums could be

1. seen
2. heard

Would resonating pounding be "seen"? or Would resonating pounding be "heard"?

The Trap of Familiarity

Don't just choose a word because you recognize it. On difficult questions, you may only recognize one or two words. The exam doesn't have "make-believe words" on it, so don't think that just because you only recognize one word means that word must be correct. If you don't recognize four words, then focus on the one that you do recognize. Is it correct? Try your best to determine if it fits the sentence. If it does, that is great, but if it doesn't, eliminate it.

Part I- Mathematics Test Review

The Mathematics Test section of the exam consists of 30 questions. They should not require anything more advanced than 8th grade level math.

Numbers and their Classifications

Numbers are the basic building blocks of mathematics. Specific features of numbers are identified by the following terms:

- Integers – The set of whole positive and negative numbers, including zero. Integers do not include fractions ($\frac{1}{3}$), decimals (0.56), or mixed numbers ($7\frac{3}{4}$).
- Prime number – A whole number greater than 1 that has only two factors, itself and 1; that is, a number that can be divided evenly only by 1 and itself.

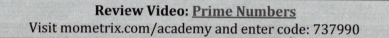

Review Video: Prime Numbers
Visit mometrix.com/academy and enter code: 737990

- Composite number – A whole number greater than 1 that has more than two different factors; in other words, any whole number that is not a prime number. For example: The composite number 8 has the factors of 1, 2, 4, and 8.
- Even number – Any integer that can be divided by 2 without leaving a remainder. For example: 2, 4, 6, 8, and so on.
- Odd number – Any integer that cannot be divided evenly by 2. For example: 3, 5, 7, 9, and so on.
- Decimal number – a number that uses a decimal point to show the part of the number that is less than one. *Example*: 1.234.
- Decimal point – a symbol used to separate the ones place from the tenths place in decimals or dollars from cents in currency.
- Decimal place – the position of a number to the right of the decimal point. In the decimal 0.123, the 1 is in the first place to the right of the decimal point, indicating tenths; the 2 is in the second place, indicating hundredths; and the 3 is in the third place, indicating thousandths.
- The decimal, or base 10, system is a number system that uses ten different digits (0, 1, 2, 3, 4, 5, 6, 7, 8, 9). An example of a number system that uses something other than ten digits is the binary, or base 2, number system, used by computers, which uses only the numbers 0 and 1. It is thought that the decimal system originated because people had only their 10 fingers for counting.

- Rational, irrational, and real numbers can be described as follows:
- Rational numbers include all integers, decimals, and fractions. Any terminating or repeating decimal number is a rational number.

- Irrational numbers cannot be written as fractions or decimals because the number of decimal places is infinite and there is no recurring pattern of digits within the number. For example, pi (π) begins with 3.141592 and continues without terminating or repeating, so pi is an irrational number.
- Real numbers are the set of all rational and irrational numbers.

Operations

There are four basic mathematical operations:

Addition increases the value of one quantity by the value of another quantity.

Example: $2 + 4 = 6; 8 + 9 = 17$. The result is called the sum. With addition, the order does not matter. $4 + 2 = 2 + 4$.

Subtraction is the opposite operation to addition; it decreases the value of one quantity by the value of another quantity.

Example: $6 - 4 = 2; 17 - 8 = 9$. The result is called the difference. Note that with subtraction, the order does matter. $6 - 4 \neq 4 - 6$.

Multiplication can be thought of as repeated addition. One number tells how many times to add the other number to itself.

Example: 3×2 (three times two) $= 2 + 2 + 2 = 6$. With multiplication, the order does not matter. $2 \times 3 = 3 \times 2$ or $3 + 3 = 2 + 2 + 2$.

Division is the opposite operation to multiplication; one number tells us how many parts to divide the other number into.

Example: $20 \div 4 = 5$; if 20 is split into 4 equal parts, each part is 5. With division, the order of the numbers does matter. $20 \div 4 \neq 4 \div 20$.

An exponent is a superscript number placed next to another number at the top right. It indicates how many times the base number is to be multiplied by itself. Exponents provide a shorthand way to write what would be a longer mathematical expression. *Example*: $a^2 = a \times a$; $2^4 = 2 \times 2 \times 2 \times 2$. A number with an exponent of 2 is said to be "squared," while a number with an exponent of 3 is said to be "cubed." The value of a number raised to an exponent is called its power. So, 8^4 is read as "8 to the 4th power," or "8 raised to the power of 4." A negative exponent is the same as the reciprocal of a positive exponent. *Example*: $a^{-2} = \frac{1}{a^2}$.

> **Review Video: Exponents**
> Visit mometrix.com/academy and enter code: 600998

Parentheses are used to designate which operations should be done first when there are multiple operations. *Example*: $4 - (2 + 1) = 1$; the parentheses tell us that we must add 2 and 1, and then subtract the sum from 4, rather than subtracting 2 from 4 and then adding 1 (this would give us an answer of 3).

> **Review Video: Mathematical Parentheses**
> Visit mometrix.com/academy and enter code: 978600

Order of Operations is a set of rules that dictates the order in which we must perform each operation in an expression so that we will evaluate it accurately. If we have an expression that includes multiple different operations, Order of Operations tells us which operations to do first. The most common mnemonic for Order of Operations is PEMDAS, or "Please Excuse My Dear Aunt Sally." PEMDAS stands for Parentheses, Exponents, Multiplication, Division, Addition, Subtraction. It is important to understand that multiplication and division have equal precedence, as do addition and subtraction, so those pairs of operations are simply worked from left to right in order.

> **Review Video: Order of Operations**
> Visit mometrix.com/academy and enter code: 259675

Example: Evaluate the expression $5 + 20 \div 4 \times (2 + 3)^2 - 6$ using the correct order of operations.

P: Perform the operations inside the parentheses, $(2 + 3) = 5$.

E: Simplify the exponents, $(5)^2 = 25$.

The equation now looks like this: $5 + 20 \div 4 \times 25 - 6$.

MD: Perform multiplication and division from left to right, $20 \div 4 = 5$; then $5 \times 25 = 125$.

The equation now looks like this: $5 + 125 - 6$.

AS: Perform addition and subtraction from left to right, $5 + 125 = 130$; then $130 - 6 = 124$.

The laws of exponents are as follows:

1. Any number to the power of 1 is equal to itself: $a^1 = a$.
2. The number 1 raised to any power is equal to 1: $1^n = 1$.
3. Any number raised to the power of 0 is equal to 1: $a^0 = 1$.

4. Add exponents to multiply powers of the same base number: $a^n \times a^m = a^{n+m}$.
5. Subtract exponents to divide powers of the same number; that is $a^n \div a^m = a^{n-m}$.
6. Multiply exponents to raise a power to a power: $(a^n)^m = a^{n \times m}$.
7. If multiplied or divided numbers inside parentheses are collectively raised to a power, this is the same as each individual term being raised to that power: $(a \times b)^n = a^n \times b^n$; $(a \div b)^n = a^n \div b^n$.

> **Review Video: Laws of Exponents**
> Visit mometrix.com/academy and enter code: 532558

Note: Exponents do not have to be integers. Fractional or decimal exponents follow all the rules above as well. *Example*: $5^{\frac{1}{4}} \times 5^{\frac{3}{4}} = 5^{\frac{1}{4}+\frac{3}{4}} = 5^1 = 5$.

A root, such as a square root, is another way of writing a fractional exponent. Instead of using a superscript, roots use the radical symbol ($\sqrt{}$) to indicate the operation. A radical will have a number underneath the bar, and may sometimes have a number in the upper left: $\sqrt[n]{a}$, read as "the nth root of a." The relationship between radical notation and exponent notation can be described by this equation: $\sqrt[n]{a} = a^{\frac{1}{n}}$. The two special cases of $n = 2$ and $n = 3$ are called square roots and cube roots. If there is no number to the upper left, it is understood to be a square root ($n = 2$). Nearly all of the roots you encounter will be square roots. A square root is the same as a number raised to the one-half power. When we say that a is the square root of b ($a = \sqrt{b}$), we mean that a multiplied by itself equals b: ($a \times a = b$).

> **Review Video: Roots**
> Visit mometrix.com/academy and enter code: 795655

A perfect square is a number that has an integer for its square root. There are 10 perfect squares from 1 to 100: 1, 4, 9, 16, 25, 36, 49, 64, 81, 100 (the squares of integers 1 through 10).

> **Review Video: Square Root and Perfect Square**
> Visit mometrix.com/academy and enter code: 648063

Scientific notation is a way of writing large numbers in a shorter form. The form $a \times 10^n$ is used in scientific notation, where a is greater than or equal to 1, but less than 10, and n is the number of places the decimal must move to get from the original number to a.

Example: The number 230,400,000 is cumbersome to write. To write the value in scientific notation, place a decimal point between the first and second numbers, and include all digits through the last non-zero digit ($a = 2.304$). To find the appropriate power of 10, count the number of places the decimal point had to move ($n = 8$). The number is positive if the decimal moved to the left, and negative if it moved to the right. We can then write 230,400,000 as 2.304×10^8.

If we look instead at the number 0.00002304, we have the same value for a, but this time the decimal moved 5 places to the right ($n = -5$). Thus, 0.00002304 can be written as 2.304×10^{-5}.

Using this notation makes it simple to compare very large or very small numbers. By comparing exponents, it is easy to see that 3.28×10^4 is smaller than 1.51×10^5, because 4 is less than 5.

Review Video: <u>Scientific Notation</u>
Visit mometrix.com/academy and enter code: 976454

Factors and Multiples

Factors are numbers that are multiplied together to obtain a product. For example, in the equation $2 \times 3 = 6$, the numbers 2 and 3 are factors. A prime number has only two factors (1 and itself), but other numbers can have many factors.

A common factor is a number that divides exactly into two or more other numbers. For example, the factors of 12 are 1, 2, 3, 4, 6, and 12, while the factors of 15 are 1, 3, 5, and 15. The common factors of 12 and 15 are 1 and 3.

A prime factor is also a prime number. Therefore, the prime factors of 12 are 2 and 3. For 15, the prime factors are 3 and 5.

The greatest common factor (GCF) is the largest number that is a factor of two or more numbers. For example, the factors of 15 are 1, 3, 5, and 15; the factors of 35 are 1, 5, 7, and 35. Therefore, the greatest common factor of 15 and 35 is 5.

Review Video: <u>Greatest Common Factor (GCF)</u>
Visit mometrix.com/academy and enter code: 838699

The least common multiple (LCM) is the smallest number that is a multiple of two or more numbers. For example, the multiples of 3 include 3, 6, 9, 12, 15, etc.; the multiples of 5 include 5, 10, 15, 20, etc. Therefore, the least common multiple of 3 and 5 is 15.

Review Video: <u>Least Common Multiple</u>
Visit mometrix.com/academy and enter code: 946579

Fractions, Percentages, and Related Concepts

A fraction is a number that is expressed as one integer written above another integer, with a dividing line between them $\left(\frac{x}{y}\right)$. It represents the quotient of the two numbers "x divided by y." It can also be thought of as x out of y equal parts.

Review Video: <u>Fractions</u>
Visit mometrix.com/academy and enter code: 262335

The top number of a fraction is called the numerator, and it represents the number of parts under consideration. The 1 in $\frac{1}{4}$ means that 1 part out of the whole is being considered in the calculation. The bottom number of a fraction is called the denominator, and it represents the total number of

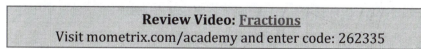

equal parts. The 4 in $\frac{1}{4}$ means that the whole consists of 4 equal parts. A fraction cannot have a denominator of zero; this is referred to as "undefined."

Fractions can be manipulated, without changing the value of the fraction, by multiplying or dividing (but not adding or subtracting) both the numerator and denominator by the same number. If you divide both numbers by a common factor, you are reducing or simplifying the fraction. Two fractions that have the same value, but are expressed differently are known as equivalent fractions. For example, $\frac{2}{10}, \frac{3}{15}, \frac{4}{20}$, and $\frac{5}{25}$ are all equivalent fractions. They can also all be reduced or simplified to $\frac{1}{5}$.

When two fractions are manipulated so that they have the same denominator, this is known as finding a common denominator. The number chosen to be that common denominator should be the least common multiple of the two original denominators. *Example:* $\frac{3}{4}$ and $\frac{5}{6}$; the least common multiple of 4 and 6 is 12. Manipulating to achieve the common denominator: $\frac{3}{4} = \frac{9}{12}; \frac{5}{6} = \frac{10}{12}$.

If two fractions have a common denominator, they can be added or subtracted simply by adding or subtracting the two numerators and retaining the same denominator. *Example:* $\frac{1}{2} + \frac{1}{4} = \frac{2}{4} + \frac{1}{4} = \frac{3}{4}$. If the two fractions do not already have the same denominator, one or both of them must be manipulated to achieve a common denominator before they can be added or subtracted.

Two fractions can be multiplied by multiplying the two numerators to find the new numerator and the two denominators to find the new denominator. *Example:* $\frac{1}{3} \times \frac{2}{3} = \frac{1 \times 2}{3 \times 3} = \frac{2}{9}$.

Two fractions can be divided flipping the numerator and denominator of the second fraction and then proceeding as though it were a multiplication. *Example:* $\frac{2}{3} \div \frac{3}{4} = \frac{2}{3} \times \frac{4}{3} = \frac{8}{9}$.

A fraction whose denominator is greater than its numerator is known as a proper fraction, while a fraction whose numerator is greater than its denominator is known as an improper fraction. Proper fractions have values less than one and improper fractions have values greater than one.

A mixed number is a number that contains both an integer and a fraction. Any improper fraction can be rewritten as a mixed number. *Example:* $\frac{8}{3} = \frac{6}{3} + \frac{2}{3} = 2 + \frac{2}{3} = 2\frac{2}{3}$. Similarly, any mixed number can be rewritten as an improper fraction. *Example:* $1\frac{3}{5} = 1 + \frac{3}{5} = \frac{5}{5} + \frac{3}{5} = \frac{8}{5}$.

Percentages can be thought of as fractions that are based on a whole of 100; that is, one whole is equal to 100%. The word percent means "per hundred." Fractions can be expressed as percents by finding equivalent fractions with a denomination of 100. *Example:* $\frac{7}{10} = \frac{70}{100} = 70\%; \frac{1}{4} = \frac{25}{100} = 25\%$.

To express a percentage as a fraction, divide the percentage number by 100 and reduce the fraction to its simplest possible terms. *Example:* $60\% = \frac{60}{100} = \frac{3}{5}; 96\% = \frac{96}{100} = \frac{24}{25}$.

Converting decimals to percentages and percentages to decimals is as simple as moving the decimal point. To convert from a decimal to a percent, move the decimal point two places to the right. To convert from a percent to a decimal, move it two places to the left. *Example*: 0.23 = 23%; 5.34 = 534%; 0.007 = 0.7%; 700% = 7.00; 86% = 0.86; 0.15% = 0.0015.

It may be helpful to remember that the percentage number will always be larger than the equivalent decimal number.

A percentage problem can be presented three main ways: (1) Find what percentage of some number another number is. *Example*: What percentage of 40 is 8? (2) Find what number is some percentage of a given number. *Example*: What number is 20% of 40? (3) Find what number another number is a given percentage of. *Example*: What number is 8 20% of? The three components in all of these cases are the same: a whole (W), a part (P), and a percentage (%). These are related by the equation: $P = W \times \%$. This is the form of the equation you would use to solve problems of type (2). To solve types (1) and (3), you would use these two forms: $\% = \frac{P}{W}$ and $W = \frac{P}{\%}$.

The thing that frequently makes percentage problems difficult is that they are most often also word problems, so a large part of solving them is figuring out which quantities are what. *Example*: In a school cafeteria, 7 students choose pizza, 9 choose hamburgers, and 4 choose tacos. Find the percentage that chooses tacos. To find the whole, you must first add all of the parts: 7 + 9 + 4 = 20. The percentage can then be found by dividing the part by the whole ($\% = \frac{P}{W}$): $\frac{4}{20} = \frac{20}{100} = 20\%$.

> **Review Video: Percentages**
> Visit mometrix.com/academy and enter code: 141911

A ratio is a comparison of two quantities in a particular order. *Example*: If there are 14 computers in a lab, and the class has 20 students, there is a student to computer ratio of 20 to 14, commonly written as 20:14. Ratios are normally reduced to their smallest whole number representation, so 20:14 would be reduced to 10:7 by dividing both sides by 2.

A proportion is a relationship between two quantities that dictates how one changes when the other changes. A direct proportion describes a relationship in which a quantity increases by a set amount for every increase in the other quantity, or decreases by that same amount for every decrease in the other quantity.

Example: Assuming a constant driving speed, the time required for a car trip increases as the distance of the trip increases. The distance to be traveled and the time required to travel are directly proportional.

Inverse proportion is a relationship in which an increase in one quantity is accompanied by a decrease in the other, or vice versa.

Example: the time required for a car trip decreases as the speed increases, and increases as the speed decreases, so the time required is inversely proportional to the speed of the car.

> **Review Video: Ratios and Percentages**
> Visit mometrix.com/academy and enter code: 904334

Part I – Form Relationship Test

The Part I Form Relationship Test requires you to visualize differences in object and manipulate things mentally.

Work Fast

The problems can be real brain teasers, because for most questions you would be able to figure out the correct answer if you had an infinite amount of time. That's why on this section more than any other you have to be conscious of time.

Rule Busters

Each problem provides you with some known information in the form of a relationship between two shapes. Look at the relationship given and decide what obvious characteristics the correct answer needs to have. These are the rules that you have to work with. Rule busters are answer choices that immediately clash with a rule and can be quickly ruled out.

Example: The given pair of shapes are both circles. The first shape in the pair that you must complete is a square, so your choice must be a square.

This is a rule. Therefore, any answer choice that is not a square is a rule buster, and is wrong! Quickly scan through the list of answer choices and eliminate all of those that are not squares.

Identify the Odd Shape

Find the most unusual feature that the correct answer needs to have, and then check the answer choices for a shape containing that feature. Don't waste time on the common features, but find the unusual feature and spend your time looking only among the answer choices that have it.

Process of Elimination

If you can't figure out which one is best, figure out which ones are worst. If you can safely eliminate certain answer choices, then you improve your chances at a guess and with the tight time restrictions you face, guessing will be an important part of your strategy on this particular test section.

Identify the Differences

What is different between the answer choices given? If all the answer choices are the same shape, don't waste time trying to figure out what shape the correct answer should be. Focus on the features that are different and then you can narrow your answer choice down to the correct answer.

Tough Questions

If you are stumped on a problem or it appears too hard or too difficult, don't waste time. Move on! Remember though, if you can quickly check for obvious "rule busters" your chances of guessing correctly are greatly improved. Before you completely give up, at least check for the easy rule busters, which should knock out a couple of possible answers. Eliminate what you can and then guess at the remainder before moving on.

Answer Selection

Eliminate choices as soon as you realize they are wrong. But be careful! Make sure you consider all of the possible answer choices. Just because one appears right, doesn't mean that the next one won't be even better! Don't worry if you are stuck between two that seem right and can't figure out which is the one. By eliminating the other choices your odds of guessing right are now 50/50 if you have it down to two. Rather than wasting too much time, play the odds. You are guessing, but guessing wisely, because you've been able to knock out some of the answer choices that you know are wrong. If you are eliminating choices and realize that the answer choice you are left with is also obviously wrong, don't panic. Start over and consider each choice again. There may easily be something that you missed the first time and will realize on the second pass.

The best way to pick an answer choice is to eliminate all of those that are wrong, until only one is left and confirm that is the correct answer and meets all of the established rules. Sometimes though, an answer choice may immediately look right. Be careful! Take a second to make sure that the other choices are not equally obvious. Don't make a hasty mistake. There are only two times that you should move on before checking other answers. First is when you are positive that the answer choice you have selected satisfies all of the rules. Second is when time is almost out and you have to make a quick guess!

Final Notes

Some problems may require that you understand a complex relationship between two shapes. Always use your time efficiently. Don't panic, stay focused. Work systematically. View the answer choices carefully. Eliminate the ones that are immediately wrong. Keep narrowing the search until you are either left with the answer or must guess at the answer from a more selective group of choices. This strategy will maximize your score on this section.

Part II – Spelling Test

It is extremely difficult to teach someone how to be a good speller, if they have been a bad speller all their life. Becoming a good speller takes lots of time. That is why we have decided to create a link review for this section of this test. Use the links listed below to work on your spelling to succeed on the test.

http://www.aaaspell.com/spelling/8

http://eslus.com/LESSONS/SPELL/SPELL.HTM

http://www.esl-lounge.com/quiz-spelling.shtml

Part III- Natural Sciences Test Review

These questions will test your knowledge of basic principles and concepts in biology, chemistry, and physics.

While a general knowledge of these subjects is important, a complete mastery of them is NOT necessary to succeed on the Science Test. Don't be intimidated by the questions presented. They do not require highly advanced knowledge, but only the ability to recognize common problem types and apply basic principles and concepts to solving them.

That is our goal, to show you the simple methods to solving these problems, so that while you will not gain a mastery of these subjects from this guide, you will learn the methods necessary to succeed on the exam.

This test may scare you. It may have been years since you've studied some of the basic concepts covered, and for even the most accomplished and studied student, these terms may be unfamiliar. General test-taking skill will help the most. DO NOT run out of time, move quickly, and use the easy pacing methods we outlined in the test-taking tactics section.

The most important thing you can do is to ignore your fears and jump into the test immediately- do not be overwhelmed by any strange-sounding terms. You have to jump into the test like jumping into a pool- all at once is the easiest way. Managing your time on this test can prove to be extremely difficult, as some of the questions may leave you stumped and countless minutes may waste away while you rack your brain for the answer. To be successful though, you must work efficiently and get through the entire test before running out of time.

Scientific Foundations

Scientific Method

One could argue that scientific knowledge is the sum of all scientific inquiries for truths about the natural world carried out throughout the history of human kind. More simply put, it is thanks to scientific inquiry that we know what we do about the world. Scientists use a number of generally accepted techniques collectively known as the scientific method. The scientific method generally involves carrying out the following steps:

- Identifying a problem or posing a question
- Formulating a hypothesis or an educated guess
- Conducting experiments or tests that will provide a basis to solve the problem or answer the question
- Observing the results of the test
- Drawing conclusions

An important part of the scientific method is using acceptable experimentation techniques to ensure results are not skewed. Objectivity is also important if valid results are to be obtained. Another important part of the scientific method is peer review. It is essential that experiments be performed and data be recorded in such a way that experiments can be reproduced to verify results.

A scientific fact is considered an objective and verifiable observation. A scientific theory is a greater body of accepted knowledge, principles, or relationships that might explain why something happens. A hypothesis is an educated guess that is not yet proven. It is used to predict the outcome of an experiment in an attempt to solve a problem or answer a question. A law is an explanation of events that always lead to the same outcome. It is a fact that an object falls. The law of gravity explains why an object falls. The theory of relativity, although generally accepted, has been neither proven nor disproved. A model is used to explain something on a smaller scale or in simpler terms to provide an example. It is a representation of an idea that can be used to explain events or applied to new situations to predict outcomes or determine results.

> **Review Video: The Scientific Method**
> Visit mometrix.com/academy and enter code: 191386

History of Science

When one examines the history of scientific knowledge, it is clear that it is constantly evolving. The body of facts, models, theories, and laws grows and changes over time. In other words, one scientific discovery leads to the next. Some advances in science and technology have important and long-lasting effects on science and society. Some discoveries were so alien to the accepted beliefs of the time that not only were they rejected as wrong, but were also considered outright blasphemy. Today, however, many beliefs once considered incorrect have become an ingrained part of scientific knowledge, and have also been the basis of new advances.

Examples of advances include: Copernicus's heliocentric view of the universe, Newton's laws of motion and planetary orbits, relativity, geologic time scale, plate tectonics, atomic theory, nuclear physics, biological evolution, germ theory, industrial revolution, molecular biology, information and communication, quantum theory, galactic universe, and medical and health technology.

Anton van Leeuwenhoek (d. 1723) used homemade magnifying glasses to become the first person to observe single-celled organisms. He observed bacteria, yeast, plants, and other microscopic organisms. His observations contributed to the field of microbiology.

Carl Linnaeus (d. 1778) created a method to classify plants and animals, which became known as the Linnaean taxonomy. This was an important contribution because it offered a way to organize and therefore study large amounts of data.

Charles Robert Darwin (d. 1882) is best known for contributing to the survival of the fittest through natural selection theory of evolution by observing different species of birds, specifically finches, in various geographic locations. Although the species Darwin looked at were different, he speculated they had a common ancestor. He reasoned that specific traits persisted because they gave the birds a greater chance of surviving and reproducing. He also discovered fossils, noted stratification, dissected marine animals, and interacted with indigenous peoples. He contributed to the fields of biology, marine biology, anthropology, paleontology, geography, and zoology.

Gregor Johann Mendel (d. 1884) is famous for experimenting with pea plants to observe the occurrence of inherited traits. He eventually became known as the father of genetics.

Barbara McClintock (d. 1992) created the first genetic map for maize and was able to demonstrate basic genetic principles, such as how recombination is an exchange of chromosomal information. She also discovered how transposition flips the switch for traits. Her work contributed to the field of genetics, in particular to areas of study concerned with the structure and function of cells and chromosomes.

James Watson and Francis Crick (d. 2004) were co-discoverers of the structure of deoxyribonucleic acid (DNA), which has a double helix shape. DNA contains the code for genetic information. The discovery of the double helix shape was important because it helped to explain how DNA replicates.

Mathematics of Science

Using the metric system is generally accepted as the preferred method for taking measurements. Having a universal standard allows individuals to interpret measurements more easily, regardless of where they are located. The basic units of measurement are: the meter, which measures length; the liter, which measures volume; and the gram, which measures mass. The metric system starts with a base unit and increases or decreases in units of 10. The prefix and the base unit combined are used to indicate an amount. For example, deka is 10 times the base unit. A dekameter is 10 meters; a dekaliter is 10 liters; and a dekagram is 10 grams. The prefix hecto refers to 100 times the base amount; kilo is 1,000 times the base amount. The prefixes that indicate a fraction of the base unit are deci, which is 1/10 of the base unit; centi, which is 1/100 of the base unit; and milli, which is 1/1000 of the base unit.

The mathematical concept of significant figures or significant digits is often used to determine the precision of measurements or the level of confidence one has in a specific measurement. The significant figures of a measurement include all the digits known with certainty plus one estimated or uncertain digit. There are a number of rules for determining which digits are considered "important" or "interesting." They are: all non-zero digits are significant, zeros between digits are significant, and leading and trailing zeros are not significant unless they appear to the right of the non-zero digits in a decimal. For example, in 0.01230 the significant digits are 1230, and this number would be said to be accurate to the hundred-thousandths place. The zero indicates that the amount has actually been measured as 0. Other zeros are considered place holders, and are not important. A decimal point may be placed after zeros to indicate their importance (in 100. for example).

Scientific notation is used because values in science can be very large or very small, which makes them unwieldy. A number in decimal notation is 93,000,000. In scientific notation, it is 9.3 x 107. The first number, 9.3, is the coefficient. It is always greater than or equal to 1 and less than 10. This number is followed by a multiplication sign. The base is always 10 in scientific notation. If the number is greater than ten, the exponent is positive. If the number is between zero and one, the exponent is negative. The first digit of the number is followed by a decimal point and then the rest of the number. In this case, the number is 9.3. To get that number, the decimal point was moved seven places from the end of the number, 93,000,000. The number of places, seven, is the exponent.

Statistics

Data collected during a science lab can be organized and presented in any number of ways. While straight narrative is a suitable method for presenting some lab results, it is not a suitable way to present numbers and quantitative measurements. These types of observations can often be better presented with tables and graphs. Data that is presented in tables and organized in rows and columns may also be used to make graphs quite easily. Other methods of presenting data include illustrations, photographs, video, and even audio formats. In a formal report, tables and figures are labeled and referred to by their labels. For example, a picture of a bubbly solution might be labeled Figure 1, Bubbly Solution. It would be referred to in the text in the following way: "The reaction created bubbles 10 mm in size, as shown in Figure 1, Bubbly Solution." Graphs are also labeled as figures. Tables are labeled in a different way. Examples include: Table 1, Results of Statistical Analysis, or Table 2, Data from Lab 2.

Graphs and charts are effective ways to present scientific data such as observations, statistical analyses, and comparisons between dependent variables and independent variables. On a line chart, the independent variable (the one that is being manipulated for the experiment) is represented on the horizontal axis (the x-axis). Any dependent variables (the ones that may change as the independent variable changes) are represented on the y-axis. The points are charted and a line is drawn to connect the points. An XY or scatter plot is often used to plot many points. A "best fit" line is drawn, which allows outliers to be identified more easily. Charts and their axes should have titles. The x and y interval units should be evenly spaced and labeled. Other types of charts are bar charts and histograms, which can be used to compare differences between the data collected for two variables. A pie chart can graphically show the relation of parts to a whole.

Mean: The mean is the sum of a list of numbers divided by the number of numbers.

Median: If there is an even number of values in the set, the median is calculated by taking the average of the two middle values.

Standard deviation: This measures the variability of a data set and determines the amount of confidence one can have in the conclusions.

Mode: This is the value that appears most frequently in a data set.

> **Review Video: Mean, Median, and Mode**
> Visit mometrix.com/academy and enter code: 286207

Range: This is the difference between the highest and lowest numbers, which can be used to determine how spread out data is.

Regression Analysis: This is a method of analyzing sets of data and sets of variables that involves studying how the typical value of the dependent variable changes when any one of the independent variables is varied and the other independent variables remain fixed.

Earth and Space Science

Geology

Minerals are naturally occurring, inorganic solids with a definite chemical composition and an orderly internal crystal structure. A polymorph is two minerals with the same chemical composition, but a different crystal structure. Rocks are aggregates of one or more minerals, and may also contain mineraloids (minerals lacking a crystalline structure) and organic remains.

The three types of rocks are sedimentary, igneous, and metamorphic. Rocks are classified based on their formation and the minerals they contain. Minerals are classified by their chemical composition. Geology is the study of the planet Earth as it pertains to the composition, structure, and origin of its rocks. Petrology is the study of rocks, including their composition, texture, structure, occurrence, mode of formation, and history. Mineralogy is the study of minerals.

> **Review Video:** Igneous, Sedimentary, and Metamorphic Rocks
> Visit mometrix.com/academy and enter code: 689294

Sedimentary rocks are formed by the process of lithification, which involves compaction, the expulsion of liquids from pores, and the cementation of the pre-existing rock. It is pressure and temperature that are responsible for this process. Sedimentary rocks are often formed in layers in the presence of water, and may contain organic remains, such as fossils. Sedimentary rocks are organized into three groups: detrital, biogenic, and chemical. Texture refers to the size, shape, and grains of sedimentary rock. Texture can be used to determine how a particular sedimentary rock was created. Composition refers to the types of minerals present in the rock. The origin of sedimentary rock refers to the type of water that was involved in its creation. Marine deposits, for example, likely involved ocean environments, while continental deposits likely involved dry land and lakes.

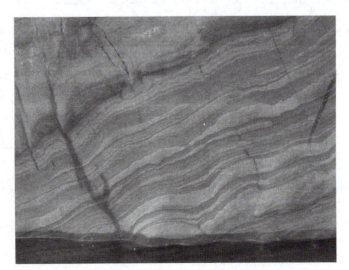

Igneous rock is formed from magma, which is molten material originating from beneath the Earth's surface. Depending upon where magma cools, the resulting igneous rock can be classified as intrusive, plutonic, hypabyssal, extrusive, or volcanic. Magma that solidifies at a depth is intrusive, cools slowly, and has a coarse grain as a result. An example is granite. Magma that solidifies at or near the surface is extrusive, cools quickly, and usually has a fine grain. An example is basalt. Magma that actually flows out of the Earth's surface is called lava. Some extrusive rock cools so quickly that crystals do not have time to form. These rocks have a glassy appearance. An example is obsidian. Hypabyssal rock is igneous rock that is formed at medium depths.

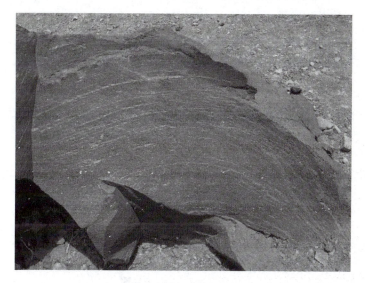

Metamorphic rock is that which has been changed by great heat and pressure. This results in a variety of outcomes, including deformation, compaction, destruction of the characteristics of the original rock, bending, folding, and formation of new minerals because of chemical reactions, and changes in the size and shape of the mineral grain. For example, the igneous rock ferromagnesian can be changed into schist and gneiss. The sedimentary rock carbonaceous can be changed into marble. The texture of metamorphic rocks can be classified as foliated and unfoliated. Foliation, or layering, occurs when rock is compressed along one axis during recrystallization. This can be seen in schist and shale. Unfoliated rock does not include this banding. Rocks that are compressed equally from all sides or lack specific minerals will be unfoliated. An example is marble.

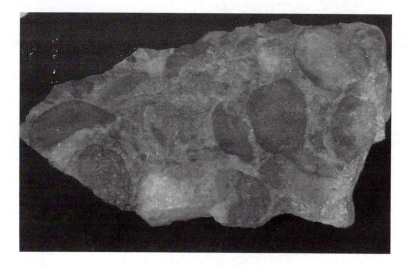

Fossils are preservations of plants, animals, their remains, or their traces that date back to about 10,000 years ago. Fossils and where they are found in rock strata makes up the fossil record. Fossils are formed under a very specific set of conditions. The fossil must not be damaged by predators and scavengers after death, and the fossil must not decompose. Usually, this happens when the organism is quickly covered with sediment. This sediment builds up and molecules in the organism's body are replaced by minerals. Fossils come in an array of sizes, from single-celled organisms to large dinosaurs.

Plate Tectonics

The Earth is ellipsoid, not perfectly spherical. This means the diameter is different through the poles and at the equator. Through the poles, the Earth is about 12,715 km in diameter. The approximate center of the Earth is at a depth of 6,378 km. The Earth is divided into a crust, mantle, and core. The core consists of a solid inner portion. Moving outward, the molten outer core occupies the space from about a depth of 5,150 km to a depth of 2,890 km. The mantle consists of a lower and upper layer. The lower layer includes the D' (D prime) and D" (D double-prime) layers. The solid portion of the upper mantle and crust together form the lithosphere, or rocky sphere. Below this, but still within the mantle, is the asthenosphere, or weak sphere. These layers are distinguishable because the lithosphere is relatively rigid, while the asthenosphere resembles a thick liquid.

The theory of plate tectonics states that the lithosphere, the solid portion of the mantle and Earth's crust, consists of major and minor plates. These plates are on top of and move with the viscous upper mantle, which is heated because of the convection cycle that occurs in the interior of the Earth. There are different estimates as to the exact number of major and minor plates. The number of major plates is believed to be between 9 and 15, and it is thought that there may be as many as 40 minor plates. The United States is atop the North American plate. The Pacific Ocean is atop the Pacific plate. The point at which these two plates slide horizontally along the San Andreas fault is an example of a transform plate boundary. The other two types of boundaries are divergent (plates that are spreading apart and forming new crust) and convergent (the process of subduction causes one plate to go under another). The movement of plates is what causes other features of the Earth's crust, such as mountains, volcanoes, and earthquakes.

> **Review Video:** Plate Tectonic Theory
> Visit mometrix.com/academy and enter code: 535013

Volcanoes can occur along any type of tectonic plate boundary. At a divergent boundary, as plates move apart, magma rises to the surface, cools, and forms a ridge. An example of this is the mid-Atlantic ridge. Convergent boundaries, where one plate slides under another, are often areas with a lot of volcanic activity. The subduction process creates magma. When it rises to the surface, volcanoes can be created. Volcanoes can also be created in the middle of a plate over hot spots. Hot spots are locations where narrow plumes of magma rise through the mantle in a fixed place over a long period of time. The Hawaiian Islands and Midway are examples. The plate shifts and the island moves. Magma continues to rise through the mantle, however, which produces another island. Volcanoes can be active, dormant, or extinct. Active volcanoes are those that are erupting or about to erupt. Dormant volcanoes are those that might erupt in the future and still have internal volcanic activity. Extinct volcanoes are those that will not erupt.

Geography

For the purposes of tracking time and location, the Earth is divided into sections with imaginary lines. Lines that run vertically around the globe through the poles are lines of longitude, sometimes called meridians. The Prime Meridian is the longitudinal reference point of 0. Longitude is measured in 15-degree increments toward the east or west. Degrees are further divided into 60 minutes, and each minute is divided into 60 seconds. Lines of latitude run horizontally around the Earth parallel to the equator, which is the 0 reference point and the widest point of the Earth. Latitude is the distance north or south from the equator, and is also measured in degrees, minutes, and seconds.

Tropic of Cancer: This is located at 23.5 degrees north. The Sun is directly overhead at noon on June 21st in the Tropic of Cancer, which marks the beginning of summer in the Northern Hemisphere.

Tropic of Capricorn: This is located at 23.5 degrees south. The Sun is directly overhead at noon on December 21st in the Tropic of Capricorn, which marks the beginning of winter in the Northern Hemisphere.

Arctic Circle: This is located at 66.5 degrees north, and marks the start of when the Sun is not visible above the horizon. This occurs on December 21st, the same day the Sun is directly over the Tropic of Capricorn.

Antarctic Circle: This is located at 66.5 degrees south, and marks the start of when the Sun is not visible above the horizon. This occurs on June 21st, which marks the beginning of winter in the Southern Hemisphere and is when the Sun is directly over the Tropic of Cancer.

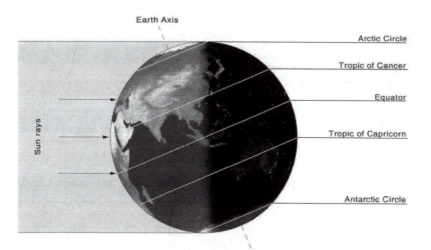

Latitude is a measurement of the distance from the equator. The distance from the equator indicates how much solar radiation a particular area receives. The equator receives more sunlight, while polar areas receive less. The Earth tilts slightly on its rotational axis. This tilt determines the seasons and affects weather. There are eight biomes or ecosystems with particular climates that are associated with latitude. Those in the high latitudes, which get the least sunlight, are tundra and taiga. Those in the mid latitudes are grassland, temperate forest, and chaparral. Those in latitudes closest to the equator are the warmest. The biomes are desert and tropical rain forest. The eighth biome is the ocean, which is unique because it consists of water and spans the entire globe. Insolation refers to incoming solar radiation. Diurnal variations refer to the daily changes in insolation. The greatest insolation occurs at noon.

The tilt of the Earth on its axis is 23.5°. This tilt causes the seasons and affects the temperature because it affects the amount of Sun the area receives. When the Northern or Southern Hemispheres are tilted toward the Sun, the hemisphere tilted toward the sun experiences summer and the other hemisphere experiences winter.

This reverses as the Earth revolves around the Sun. Fall and spring occur between the two extremes. The equator gets the same amount of sunlight every day of the year, about 12 hours, and doesn't experience seasons. Both poles have days during the winter when they are tilted away from the Sun and receive no daylight. The opposite effect occurs during the summer. There are 24 hours of daylight and no night. The summer solstice, the day with the most amount of sunlight, occurs on June 21st in the Northern Hemisphere and on December 21st in the Southern Hemisphere. The winter solstice, the day with the least amount of sunlight, occurs on December 21st in the Northern Hemisphere and on June 21st in the Southern Hemisphere.

Weather, Atmosphere, Water Cycle

Meteorology is the study of the atmosphere, particularly as it pertains to forecasting the weather and understanding its processes. Weather is the condition of the atmosphere at any given moment. Most weather occurs in the troposphere. Weather includes changing events such as clouds, storms, and temperature, as well as more extreme events such as tornadoes, hurricanes, and blizzards. Climate refers to the average weather for a particular area over time, typically at least 30 years. Latitude is an indicator of climate. Changes in climate occur over long time periods.

> **Review Video: Climate and Weather**
> Visit mometrix.com/academy and enter code: 455373

The hydrologic, or water, cycle refers to water movement on, above, and in the Earth. Water can be in any one of its three states during different phases of the cycle. The three states of water are liquid water, frozen ice, and water vapor. Processes involved in the hydrologic cycle include precipitation, canopy interception, snow melt, runoff, infiltration, subsurface flow, evaporation, sublimation, advection, condensation, and transpiration. Precipitation is when condensed water vapor falls to Earth. Examples include rain, fog drip, and various forms of snow, hail, and sleet. Canopy interception is when precipitation lands on plant foliage instead of falling to the ground and evaporating. Snow melt is runoff produced by melting snow. Infiltration occurs when water flows from the surface into the ground. Subsurface flow refers to water that flows underground. Evaporation is when water in a liquid state changes to a gas. Sublimation is when water in a solid state (such as snow or ice) changes to water vapor without going through a liquid phase. Advection

- 38 -

is the movement of water through the atmosphere. Condensation is when water vapor changes to liquid water. Transpiration is when water vapor is released from plants into the air.

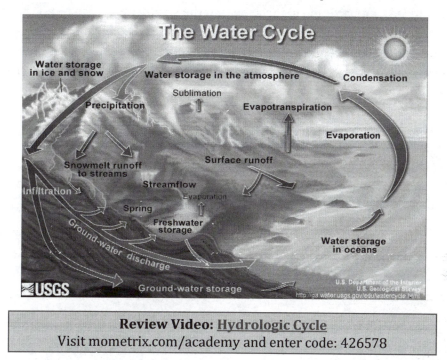

Review Video: Hydrologic Cycle
Visit mometrix.com/academy and enter code: 426578

The ocean is the salty body of water that encompasses the Earth. It has a mass of 1.4×10^{24} grams. Geographically, the ocean is divided into three large oceans: the Pacific Ocean, the Atlantic Ocean, and the Indian Ocean. There are also other divisions, such as gulfs, bays, and various types of seas, including Mediterranean and marginal seas. Ocean distances can be measured by latitude, longitude, degrees, meters, miles, and nautical miles. The ocean accounts for 70.8% of the surface of the Earth, amounting to $361,254,000$ km². The ocean's depth is greatest at Challenger Deep in the Mariana Trench. The ocean floor here is 10,924 meters below sea level. The depths of the ocean are mapped by echo sounders and satellite altimeter systems. Echo sounders emit a sound pulse from the surface and record the time it takes to return. Satellite altimeters provide better maps of the ocean floor.

The atmosphere consists of 78% nitrogen, 21% oxygen, and 1% argon. It also includes traces of water vapor, carbon dioxide and other gases, dust particles, and chemicals from Earth. The atmosphere becomes thinner the farther it is from the Earth's surface. It becomes difficult to breathe at about 3 km above sea level. The atmosphere gradually fades into space. The lowest layer of the atmosphere is called the troposphere. Its thickness varies at the poles and the equator, varying from about 7 to 17 km. This is where most weather occurs. The stratosphere is next, and continues to an elevation of about 51 km. The mesosphere extends from the stratosphere to an elevation of about 81 km. It is the coldest layer and is where meteors tend to ablate. The next layer is the thermosphere. It is where the International Space Station orbits. The exosphere is the outermost layer, extends to 10,000 km, and mainly consists of hydrogen and helium.

Earth's atmosphere has five main layers. From lowest to highest, these are the troposphere, the stratosphere, the mesosphere, the thermosphere, and the exosphere. Between each pair of layers is a transition layer called a pause. The troposphere includes the tropopause, which is the transitional layer of the stratosphere. Energy from Earth's surface is transferred to the troposphere. Temperature decreases with altitude in this layer. In the stratosphere, the temperature is inverted, meaning that it increases with altitude. The stratosphere includes the ozone layer, which helps block ultraviolet light from the Sun. The stratopause is the transitional layer to the mesosphere. The temperature of the mesosphere decreases with height. It is considered the coldest place on Earth, and has an average temperature of -85 degrees Celsius. Temperature increases with altitude in the thermosphere, which includes the thermopause. Just past the thermosphere is the exobase, the base layer of the exosphere. Beyond the five main layers are the ionosphere, homosphere, heterosphere, and magnetosphere.

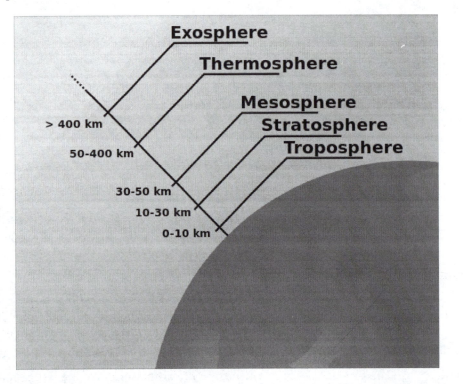

Most clouds can be classified according to the altitude of their base above Earth's surface. High clouds occur at altitudes between 5,000 and 13,000 meters. Middle clouds occur at altitudes between 2,000 and 7,000 meters. Low clouds occur from the Earth's surface to altitudes of 2,000 meters. Types of high clouds include cirrus (Ci), thin wispy mare's tails that consist of ice; cirrocumulus (Cc), small, pillow-like puffs that often appear in rows; and cirrostratus (Cs), thin, sheetlike clouds that often cover the entire sky. Types of middle clouds include altocumulus (Ac), gray-white clouds that consist of liquid water; and altostratus (As), grayish or blue-gray clouds that span the sky. Types of low clouds include stratus (St), gray and fog-like clouds consisting of water droplets that take up the whole sky; stratocumulus (Sc), low-lying, lumpy gray clouds; and nimbostratus (Ns), dark gray clouds with uneven bases that indicate rain or snow. Two types of clouds, cumulus (Cu) and cumulonimbus (Cb), are capable of great vertical growth. They can start at a wide range of altitudes, from the Earth's surface to altitudes of 13,000 meters.

Review Video: Clouds
Visit mometrix.com/academy and enter code: 803166

- 40 -

Astronomy

Astronomy is the scientific study of celestial objects and their positions, movements, and structures. Celestial does not refer to the Earth in particular, but does include its motions as it moves through space. Other objects include the Sun, the Moon, planets, satellites, asteroids, meteors, comets, stars, galaxies, the universe, and other space phenomena. The term astronomy has its roots in the Greek words "astro" and "nomos," which means "laws of the stars."

What can be seen of the universe is believed to be at least 93 billion light years across. To put this into perspective, the Milky Way galaxy is about 100,000 light years across. Our view of matter in the universe is that it forms into clumps. Matter is organized into stars, galaxies, clusters of galaxies, superclusters, and the Great Wall of galaxies. Galaxies consist of stars, some with planetary systems. Some estimates state that the universe is about 13 billion years old. It is not considered dense, and is believed to consist of 73 percent dark energy, 23 percent cold dark matter, and 4 percent regular matter. Cosmology is the study of the universe. Interstellar medium (ISM) is the gas and dust in the interstellar space between a galaxy's stars.

The solar system is a planetary system of objects that exist in an ecliptic plane. Objects orbit around and are bound by gravity to a star called the Sun. Objects that orbit around the Sun include: planets, dwarf planets, moons, asteroids, meteoroids, cosmic dust, and comets. The definition of planets has changed. At one time, there were nine planets in the solar system. There are now eight. Planetary objects in the solar system include four inner, terrestrial planets: Mercury, Venus, Earth, and Mars. They are relatively small, dense, rocky, lack rings, and have few or no moons. The four outer, or Jovian, planets are Jupiter, Saturn, Uranus, and Neptune, which are large and have low densities, rings, and moons. They are also known as gas giants. Between the inner and outer planets is the asteroid belt. Beyond Neptune is the Kuiper belt. Within these belts are five dwarf planets: Ceres, Pluto, Haumea, Makemake, and Eris.

The Sun is at the center of the solar system. It is composed of 70% hydrogen (H) and 28% helium (He). The remaining 2% is made up of metals. The Sun is one of 100 billion stars in the Milky Way galaxy. Its diameter is 1,390,000 km, its mass is 1.989×10^{30} kg, its surface temperature is 5,800 K, and its core temperature is 15,600,000 K. The Sun represents more than 99.8% of the total mass of the solar system. At the core, the temperature is 15.6 million K, the pressure is 250 billion atmospheres, and the density is more than 150 times that of water. The surface is called the photosphere. The chromosphere lies above this, and the corona, which extends millions of kilometers into space, is next. Sunspots are relatively cool regions on the surface with a temperature of 3,800 K. Temperatures in the corona are over 1,000,000 K. Its magnetosphere, or heliosphere, extends far beyond Pluto.

Mercury: Mercury is the closest to the Sun and is also the smallest planet. It orbits the Sun every 88 days, has no satellites or atmosphere, has a Moon-like surface with craters, appears bright, and is dense and rocky with a large iron core.

Venus: Venus is the second planet from the Sun. It orbits the Sun every 225 days, is very bright, and is similar to Earth in size, gravity, and bulk composition. It has a dense atmosphere composed of carbon dioxide and some sulfur. It is covered with reflective clouds made of sulfuric acid and exhibits signs of volcanism. Lightning and thunder have been recorded on Venus's surface.

Earth: Earth is the third planet from the Sun. It orbits the Sun every 365 days. Approximately 71% of its surface is salt-water oceans. The Earth is rocky, has an atmosphere composed mainly of oxygen and nitrogen, has one moon, and supports millions of species. It contains the only known life in the solar system.

Mars: Mars it the fourth planet from the Sun. It appears reddish due to iron oxide on the surface, has a thin atmosphere, has a rotational period similar to Earth's, and has seasonal cycles. Surface features of Mars include volcanoes, valleys, deserts, and polar ice caps. Mars has impact craters and the tallest mountain, largest canyon, and perhaps the largest impact crater yet discovered.

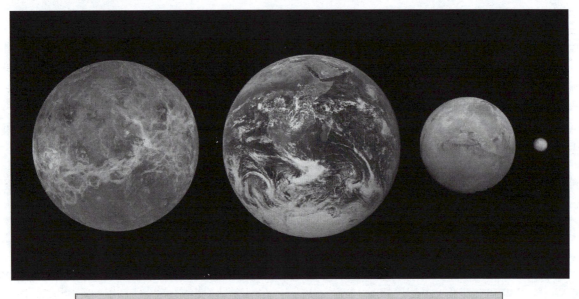

Review Video: The Inner Planets of Our Solar System
Visit mometrix.com/academy and enter code: 103427

Jupiter: Jupiter is the fifth planet from the Sun and the largest planet in the solar system. It consists mainly of hydrogen, and 25% of its mass is made up of helium. It has a fast rotation and has clouds in the tropopause composed of ammonia crystals that are arranged into bands sub-divided into lighter-hued zones and darker belts causing storms and turbulence. Jupiter has wind speeds of 100 m/s, a planetary ring, 63 moons, and a Great Red Spot, which is an anticyclonic storm.

Saturn: Saturn is the sixth planet from the Sun and the second largest planet in the solar system. It is composed of hydrogen, some helium, and trace elements. Saturn has a small core of rock and ice, a thick layer of metallic hydrogen, a gaseous outer layer, wind speeds of up to 1,800 km/h, a system of rings, and 61 moons.

Uranus: Uranus is the seventh planet from the Sun. Its atmosphere is composed mainly of hydrogen and helium, and also contains water, ammonia, methane, and traces of hydrocarbons. With a minimum temperature of 49 K, Uranus has the coldest atmosphere. Uranus has a ring system, a magnetosphere, and 13 moons.

Neptune: Neptune is the eighth planet from the Sun and is the planet with the third largest mass. It has 12 moons, an atmosphere similar to Uranus, a Great Dark Spot, and the strongest sustained winds of any planet (wind speeds can be as high as 2,100 km/h). Neptune is cold (about 55 K) and has a fragmented ring system.

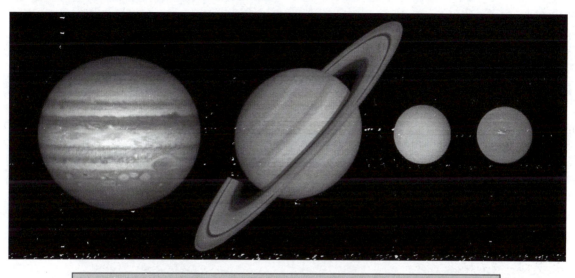

Review Video: The Outer Planets of Our Solar System
Visit mometrix.com/academy and enter code: 683995

The Earth is about 12,765 km (7,934 miles) in diameter. The Moon is about 3,476 km (2,160 mi) in diameter. The distance between the Earth and the Moon is about 384,401 km (238,910 mi). The diameter of the Sun is approximately 1,390,000 km (866,000 mi). The distance from the Earth to the Sun is 149,598,000 km, also known as 1 Astronomical Unit (AU).

The star that is nearest to the solar system is Proxima Centauri. It is about 270,000 AU away. Some distant galaxies are so far away that their light takes several billion years to reach the Earth. In other words, people on Earth see them as they looked billions of years ago.

It takes about one month for the Moon to go through all its phases. Waxing refers to the two weeks during which the Moon goes from a new moon to a full moon. About two weeks is spent waning, going from a full moon to a new moon. The lit part of the Moon always faces the Sun.

The phases of waxing are: new moon, during which the Moon is not illuminated and rises and sets with the Sun; crescent moon, during which a tiny sliver is lit; first quarter, during which half the Moon is lit and the phase of the Moon is due south on the meridian; gibbous, during which more than half of the Moon is lit and has a shape similar to a football; right side, during which the Moon is lit; and full moon, during which the Moon is fully illuminated, rises at sunset, and sets at sunrise.

After a full moon, the Moon is waning. The phases of waning are: gibbous, during which the left side is lit and the Moon rises after sunset and sets after sunrise; third quarter, during which the Moon is half lit and rises at midnight and sets at noon; crescent, during which a tiny sliver is lit; and new moon, during which the Moon is not illuminated and rises and sets with the Sun.

Biology

Cells

The main difference between eukaryotic and prokaryotic cells is that eukaryotic cells have a nucleus and prokaryotic cells do not. Eukaryotic cells are considered more complex, while prokaryotic cells are smaller and simpler. Eukaryotic cells have membrane-bound organelles that perform various functions and contribute to the complexity of these types of cells. Prokaryotic cells do not contain membrane-bound organelles. In prokaryotic cells, the genetic material (DNA) is not contained within a membrane-bound nucleus. Instead, it aggregates in the cytoplasm in a nucleoid. In eukaryotic cells, DNA is mostly contained in chromosomes in the nucleus, although there is some DNA in mitochondria and chloroplasts. Prokaryotic cells usually divide by binary fission and are haploid. Eukaryotic cells divide by mitosis and are diploid. Prokaryotic structures include plasmids, ribosomes, cytoplasm, a cytoskeleton, granules of nutritional substances, a plasma membrane, flagella, and a few others. They are single-celled organisms. Bacteria are prokaryotic cells.

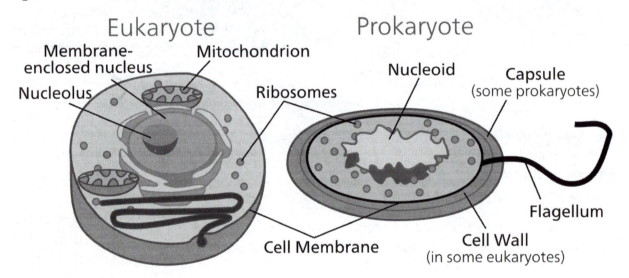

The functions of plant and animal cells vary greatly, and the functions of different cells within a single organism can also be vastly different. Animal and plant cells are similar in structure in that they are eukaryotic, which means they contain a nucleus. The nucleus is a round structure that controls the activities of the cell and contains chromosomes. Both types of cells have cell membranes, cytoplasm, vacuoles, and other structures. The main difference between the two is that plant cells have a cell wall made of cellulose that can handle high levels of pressure within the cell, which can occur when liquid enters a plant cell. Plant cells have chloroplasts that are used during the process of photosynthesis, which is the conversion of sunlight into food. Plant cells usually have

- 44 -

one large vacuole, whereas animal cells can have many smaller ones. Plant cells have a regular shape, while the shapes of animal cell can vary.

Review Video: Plant and Animal Cells
Visit mometrix.com/academy and enter code: 115568

Plant cells can be much larger than animal cells, ranging from 10 to 100 micrometers. Animal cells are 10 to 30 micrometers in size. Plant cells can have much larger vacuoles that occupy a large portion of the cell. They also have cell walls, which are thick barriers consisting of protein and sugars. Animal cells lack cell walls. Chloroplasts in plants that perform photosynthesis absorb sunlight and convert it into energy. Mitochondria produce energy from food in animal cells. Plant and animal cells are both eukaryotic, meaning they contain a nucleus. Both plant and animal cells duplicate genetic material, separate it, and then divide in half to reproduce. Plant cells build a cell plate between the two new cells, while animal cells make a cleavage furrow and pinch in half. Microtubules are components of the cytoskeleton in both plant and animal cells. Microtubule organizing centers (MTOCs) make microtubules in plant cells, while centrioles make microtubules in animal cells.

Photosynthesis is the conversion of sunlight into energy in plant cells, and also occurs in some types of bacteria and protists. Carbon dioxide and water are converted into glucose during photosynthesis, and light is required during this process. Cyanobacteria are thought to be the descendants of the first organisms to use photosynthesis about 3.5 billion years ago. Photosynthesis is a form of cellular respiration. It occurs in chloroplasts that use thylakoids, which are structures in the membrane that contain light reaction chemicals. Chlorophyll is a pigment that absorbs light. During the process, water is used and oxygen is released. The equation for the chemical reaction that occurs during photosynthesis is $6H_2O + 6CO_2 \rightarrow C_6H_{12}O_6 + 6O_2$. During photosynthesis, six molecules of water and six molecules of carbon dioxide react to form one molecule of sugar and six molecules of oxygen.

Review Video: Photosynthesis
Visit mometrix.com/academy and enter code: 227035

The term cell cycle refers to the process by which a cell reproduces, which involves cell growth, the duplication of genetic material, and cell division. Complex organisms with many cells use the cell cycle to replace cells as they lose their functionality and wear out. The entire cell cycle in animal cells can take 24 hours. The time required varies among different cell types. Human skin cells, for example, are constantly reproducing. Some other cells only divide infrequently. Once neurons are mature, they do not grow or divide. The two ways that cells can reproduce are through meiosis and mitosis. When cells replicate through mitosis, the "daughter cell" is an exact replica of the parent cell. When cells divide through meiosis, the daughter cells have different genetic coding than the parent cell. Meiosis only happens in specialized reproductive cells called gametes.

Mitosis is the process of cell reproduction in which a eukaryotic cell splits into two separate, but completely identical, cells. This process is divided into a number of different phases.

Review Video: Mitosis
Visit mometrix.com/academy and enter code: 849894

Interphase: The cell prepares for division by replicating its genetic and cytoplasmic material. Interphase can be further divided into G1, S, and G2.

Prophase: The chromatin thickens into chromosomes and the nuclear membrane begins to disintegrate. Pairs of centrioles move to opposite sides of the cell and spindle fibers begin to form. The mitotic spindle, formed from cytoskeleton parts, moves chromosomes around within the cell.

Metaphase: The spindle moves to the center of the cell and chromosome pairs align along the center of the spindle structure.

Anaphase: The pairs of chromosomes, called sisters, begin to pull apart, and may bend. When they are separated, they are called daughter chromosomes. Grooves appear in the cell membrane.

Telophase: The spindle disintegrates, the nuclear membranes reform, and the chromosomes revert to chromatin. In animal cells, the membrane is pinched. In plant cells, a new cell wall begins to form.

Cytokinesis: This is the physical splitting of the cell (including the cytoplasm) into two cells. Some believe this occurs following telophase. Others say it occurs from anaphase, as the cell begins to furrow, through telophase, when the cell actually splits into two.

Meiosis is another process by which eukaryotic cells reproduce. However, meiosis is used by more complex life forms such as plants and animals and results in four unique cells rather than two identical cells as in mitosis. Meiosis has the same phases as mitosis, but they happen twice. In addition, different events occur during some phases of meiosis than mitosis. The events that occur during the first phase of meiosis are interphase (I), prophase (I), metaphase (I), anaphase (I), telophase (I), and cytokinesis (I). During this first phase of meiosis, chromosomes cross over, genetic material is exchanged, and tetrads of four chromatids are formed. The nuclear membrane dissolves. Homologous pairs of chromatids are separated and travel to different poles. At this point, there has been one cell division resulting in two cells. Each cell goes through a second cell division, which consists of prophase (II), metaphase (II), anaphase (II), telophase (II), and cytokinesis (II). The result is four daughter cells with different sets of chromosomes. The daughter cells are haploid, which means they contain half the genetic material of the parent cell. The second phase of meiosis is similar to the process of mitosis. Meiosis encourages genetic diversity.

> **Review Video: Meiosis**
> Visit mometrix.com/academy and enter code: 247334

Genetics

Chromosomes consist of genes, which are single units of genetic information. Genes are made up of deoxyribonucleic acid (DNA). DNA is a nucleic acid located in the cell nucleus. There is also DNA in the mitochondria. DNA replicates to pass on genetic information. The DNA in almost all cells is the same. It is also involved in the biosynthesis of proteins. The model or structure of DNA is described as a double helix. A helix is a curve, and a double helix is two congruent curves connected by horizontal members. The model can be likened to a spiral staircase. It is right-handed. The British scientist Rosalind Elsie Franklin is credited with taking the x-ray diffraction image in 1952 that was used by Francis Crick and James Watson to formulate the double-helix model of DNA and speculate about its important role in carrying and transferring genetic information.

DNA has a double helix shape, resembles a twisted ladder, and is compact. It consists of nucleotides. Nucleotides consist of a five-carbon sugar (pentose), a phosphate group, and a nitrogenous base. Two bases pair up to form the rungs of the ladder. The "side rails" or backbone consists of the covalently bonded sugar and phosphate. The bases are attached to each other with hydrogen bonds, which are easily dismantled so replication can occur. Each base is attached to a phosphate and to a sugar. There are four types of nitrogenous bases: adenine (A), guanine (G), cytosine (C), and thymine (T). There are about 3 billion bases in human DNA. The bases are mostly the same in everybody, but their order is different. It is the order of these bases that creates diversity in people. Adenine (A) pairs with thymine (T), and cytosine (C) pairs with guanine (G).

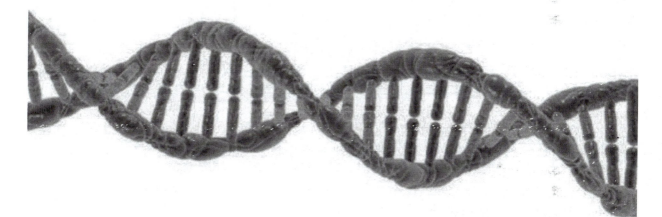

A gene is a portion of DNA that identifies how traits are expressed and passed on in an organism. A gene is part of the genetic code. Collectively, all genes form the genotype of an individual. The genotype includes genes that may not be expressed, such as recessive genes. The phenotype is the physical, visual manifestation of genes. It is determined by the basic genetic information and how genes have been affected by their environment. An allele is a variation of a gene. Also known as a trait, it determines the manifestation of a gene. This manifestation results in a specific physical appearance of some facet of an organism, such as eye color or height. For example the genetic information for eye color is a gene. The gene variations responsible for blue, green, brown, or black eyes are called alleles. Locus (pl. loci) refers to the location of a gene or alleles.

Mendel's laws are the law of segregation (the first law) and the law of independent assortment (the second law). The law of segregation states that there are two alleles and that half of the total number of alleles are contributed by each parent organism. The law of independent assortment states that traits are passed on randomly and are not influenced by other traits. The exception to this is linked traits. A Punnett square can illustrate how alleles combine from the contributing genes to form various phenotypes. One set of a parent's genes are put in columns, while the genes from the other parent are placed in rows. The allele combinations are shown in each cell. When two different alleles are present in a pair, the dominant one is expressed. A Punnett square can be used to predict the outcome of crosses.

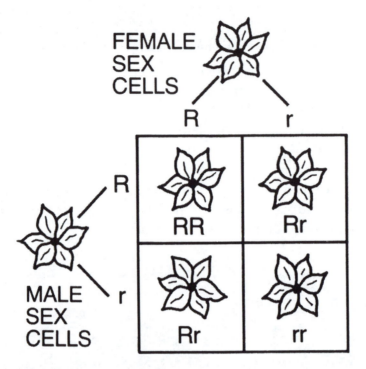

Gene traits are represented in pairs with an upper case letter for the dominant trait (A) and a lower case letter for the recessive trait (a). Genes occur in pairs (AA, Aa, or aa). There is one gene on each chromosome half supplied by each parent organism. Since half the genetic material is from each parent, the offspring's traits are represented as a combination of these. A dominant trait only requires one gene of a gene pair for it to be expressed in a phenotype, whereas a recessive requires both genes in order to be manifested. For example, if the mother's genotype is Dd and the father's is dd, the possible combinations are Dd and dd. The dominant trait will be manifested if the genotype is DD or Dd. The recessive trait will be manifested if the genotype is dd. Both DD and dd are homozygous pairs. Dd is heterozygous.

Evolution

Scientific evidence supporting the theory of evolution can be found in biogeography, comparative anatomy and embryology, the fossil record, and molecular evidence. Biogeography studies the geographical distribution of animals and plants. Evidence of evolution related to the area of biogeography includes species that are well suited for extreme environments. The fossil record shows that species lived only for a short time period before becoming extinct. The fossil record can also show the succession of plants and animals. Living fossils are existing species that have not changed much morphologically and are very similar to ancient examples in the fossil record. Examples include the horseshoe crab and gingko. Comparative embryology studies how species are similar in the embryonic stage, but become increasingly specialized and diverse as they age. Vestigial organs are those that still exist, but become nonfunctional. Examples include the hind limbs of whales and the wings of birds that can no longer fly, such as ostriches.

- 48 -

The rate of evolution is affected by the variability of a population. Variability increases the likelihood of evolution. Variability in a population can be increased by mutations, immigration, sexual reproduction (as opposed to asexual reproduction), and size. Natural selection, emigration, and smaller populations can lead to decreased variability. Sexual selection affects evolution. If fewer genes are available, it will limit the number of genes passed on to subsequent generations. Some animal mating behaviors are not as successful as others. A male that does not attract a female because of a weak mating call or dull feathers, for example, will not pass on its genes. Mechanical isolation, which refers to sex organs that do not fit together very well, can also decrease successful mating.

Natural selection: This theory developed by Darwin states that traits that help give a species a survival advantage are passed on to subsequent generations. Members of a species that do not have the advantageous trait die before they reproduce. Darwin's four principles are: from generation to generation, there are various individuals within a species; genes determine variations; more individuals are born than survive to maturation; and specific genes enable an organism to better survive.

Gradualism: This can be contrasted with punctuationism. It is an idea that evolution proceeds at a steady pace and does not include sudden developments of new species or features from one generation to the next.

Punctuated Equilibrium: This can be contrasted with gradualism. It is the idea in evolutionary biology that states that evolution involves long time periods of no change (stasis) accompanied by relatively brief periods (hundreds of thousands of years) of rapid change.

> **Review Video:** <u>**Phyletic Gradualism and Punctuated Equillibrium**</u>
> Visit mometrix.com/academy and enter code: 866012

Three types of evolution are divergent, convergent, and parallel. Divergent evolution refers to two species that become different over time. This can be caused by one of the species adapting to a different environment. Convergent evolution refers to two species that start out fairly different, but evolve to share many similar traits. Parallel evolution refers to species that are not similar and do not become more or less similar over time. Mechanisms of evolution include descent (the passing on of genetic information), mutation, migration, natural selection, and genetic variation and drift. The biological definition of species refers to a group of individuals that can mate and reproduce. Speciation refers to the evolution of a new biological species. The biological species concept (BSC) basically states that a species is a community of individuals that can reproduce and have a niche in nature.

One theory of how life originated on Earth is that life developed from nonliving materials. The first stage of this transformation happened when abiotic (nonliving) synthesis took place, which is the formation of monomers like amino acids and nucleotides. Next, monomers joined together to create polymers such as proteins and nucleic acids. These polymers are then believed to have formed into protobionts. The last stage was the development of the process of heredity. Supporters of this theory believe that RNA was the first genetic material. Another theory postulates that hereditary systems came about before the origination of nucleic acids. Another theory is that life, or the precursors for it, were transported to Earth from a meteorite or other object from space. There is no real evidence to support this theory.

A number of scientists have made significant contributions to the theory of evolution:

Cuvier (1744-1829): Cuvier was a French naturalist who used the fossil record (paleontology) to compare the anatomies of extinct species and existing species to make conclusions about extinction. He believed in the catastrophism theory more strongly than the theory of evolution.

Lamarck (1769-1832): Lamarck was a French naturalist who believed in the idea of evolution and thought it was a natural occurrence influenced by the environment. He studied medicine and botany. Lamarck put forth a theory of evolution by inheritance of acquired characteristics. He theorized that organisms became more complex by moving up a ladder of progress.

Lyell (1797-1875): Lyell was a British geologist who believed in geographical uniformitarianism, which can be contrasted with catastrophism.

Charles Robert Darwin (1809-1882): Darwin was an English naturalist known for his belief that evolution occurred by natural selection. He believed that species descend from common ancestors.

Alfred Russell Wallace (1823-1913): He was a British naturalist who independently developed a theory of evolution by natural selection. He believed in the transmutation of species (that one species develops into another).

Organism Classification

The groupings in the five kingdom classification system are kingdom, phylum/division, class, order, family, genus, and species. A memory aid for this is: King Phillip Came Over For Good Soup. The five kingdoms are Monera, Protista, Fungi, Plantae, and Animalia. The kingdom is the top level classification in this system. Below that are the following groupings: phylum, class, order, family, genus, and species. The Monera kingdom includes about 10,000 known species of prokaryotes, such as bacteria and cyanobacteria. Members of this kingdom can be unicellular organisms or colonies. The next four kingdoms consist of eukaryotes. The Protista kingdom includes about 250,000 species of unicellular protozoans and unicellular and multicellular algae. The Fungi kingdom includes about 100,000 species. A recently introduced system of classification includes a three domain grouping above kingdom. The domain groupings are Archaea, Bacteria (which both consist of prokaryotes), and Eukarya, which include eukaryotes. According to the five kingdom classification system, humans are: kingdom Animalia, phylum Chordata, subphylum Vertebrata, class Mammalia, order Primate, family Hominidae, genus Homo, and species Sapiens.

An organism is a living thing. A unicellular organism is an organism that has only one cell. Examples of unicellular organisms are bacteria and paramecium. A multicellular organism is one that consists of many cells. Humans are a good example. By some estimates, the human body is made up of billions of cells. Others think the human body has more than 75 trillion cells. The term microbe refers to small organisms that are only visible through a microscope. Examples include viruses, bacteria, fungi, and protozoa. Microbes are also referred to as microorganisms, and it is these that are studied by microbiologists. Bacteria can be rod shaped, round (cocci), or spiral (spirilla). These shapes are used to differentiate among types of bacteria. Bacteria can be identified by staining them. This particular type of stain is called a gram stain. If bacteria are gram-positive, they absorb the stain and become purple. If bacteria are gram-negative, they do not absorb the stain and become a pinkish color.

Organisms in the Protista kingdom are classified according to their methods of locomotion, their methods of reproduction, and how they get their nutrients. Protists can move by the use of a flagellum, cilia, or pseudopod. Flagellates have flagellum, which are long tails or whip-like structures that are rotated to help the protist move. Ciliates use cilia, which are smaller hair-like structures on the exterior of a cell that wiggle to help move the surrounding matter. Amoeboids use pseudopodia to move. Bacteria reproduce either sexually or asexually. Binary fission is a form of asexual reproduction whereby bacteria divide in half to produce two new organisms that are clones of the parent. In sexual reproduction, genetic material is exchanged. When kingdom members are categorized according to how they obtain nutrients, the three types of protists are photosynthetic, consumers, and saprophytes. Photosynthetic protists convert sunlight into energy. Organisms that use photosynthesis are considered producers. Consumers, also known as heterotrophs, eat or consume other organisms. Saprophytes consume dead or decaying substances.

Mycology is the study of fungi. The Fungi kingdom includes about 100,000 species. They are further delineated as mushrooms, yeasts, molds, rusts, mildews, stinkhorns, puffballs, and truffles. Fungi are characterized by cell walls that have chitin, a long chain polymer carbohydrate. Fungi are different from species in the Plant kingdom, which have cell walls consisting of cellulose. Fungi are thought to have evolved from a single ancestor. Although they are often thought of as a type of plant, they are more similar to animals than plants. Fungi are typically small and numerous, and have a diverse morphology among species. They can have bright red cups and be orange jellylike masses, and their shapes can resemble golf balls, bird nests with eggs, starfish, parasols, and male genitalia. Some members of the stinkhorn family emit odors similar to dog scat to attract flies that help transport spores that are involved in reproduction. Fungi of this family are also consumed by humans.

> **Review Video: Kingdom Fungi**
> Visit mometrix.com/academy and enter code: 315081

Chlorophyta are green algae. Bryophyta are nonvascular mosses and liverworts. They have root-like parts called rhizoids. Since they do not have the vascular structures to transport water, they live in moist environments. Lycophyta are club mosses. They are vascular plants. They use spores and need water to reproduce. Equisetopsida (sphenophyta) are horsetails. Like lycophyta, they need water to reproduce with spores. They have rhizoids and needle-like leaves. The pteridophytes (filicopsida) are ferns. They have stems (rhizomes). Spermatopsida are the seed plants. Gymnosperms are a conifer, which means they have cones with seeds that are used in reproduction. Plants with seeds require less water. Cycadophyta are cone-bearing and look like palms. Gnetophyta are plants that live in the desert. Coniferophyta are pine trees, and have both cones and needles. Ginkgophyta are ginkos. Anthophyta is the division with the largest number of plant species, and includes flowering plants with true seeds. Only plants in the division bryophyta (mosses and liverworts) are nonvascular, which means they do not have xylem to transport water. All of the plants in the remaining divisions are vascular, meaning they have true roots, stems, leaves, and xylem. Pteridophytes are plants that use spores and not seeds to reproduce. They include the following divisions: Psilophyta (whisk fern), Lycophyta (club mosses), Sphenophyta (horsetails), and Pterophyta (ferns). Spermatophytes are plants that use seeds to reproduce. Included in this category are gymnosperms, which are flowerless plants that use naked seeds, and angiosperms, which are flowering plants that contain seeds in or on a fruit. Gymnosperms include the following divisions: cycadophyta (cycads), ginkgophyta (maidenhair tree), gnetophyta (ephedra and welwitschia), and coniferophyta (which includes pinophyta conifers). Angiosperms comprise the division anthophyta (flowering plants). Plants are autotrophs, which mean they make their own food. In a sense, they are self sufficient. Three major processes used by plants are photosynthesis, transpiration, and respiration. Photosynthesis involves using sunlight to make food for plants. Transpiration evaporates water out of plants. Respiration is the utilization of food that was produced during photosynthesis.

Two major systems in plants are the shoot and the root system. The shoot system includes leaves, buds, and stems. It also includes the flowers and fruits in flowering plants. The shoot system is located above the ground. The root system is the component of the plant that is underground, and includes roots, tubers, and rhizomes. Meristems form plant cells by mitosis. Cells then differentiate into cell types to form the three types of plant tissues, which are dermal, ground, and vascular. Dermal refers to tissues that form the covering or outer layer of a plant. Ground tissues consist of parenchyma, collenchyma, and/or sclerenchyma cells.

There are at least 230,000 species of flowering plants. They represent about 90 percent of all plants. Angiosperms have a sexual reproduction phase that includes flowering. When growing plants, one may think they develop in the following order: seeds, growth, flowers, and fruit. The reproductive cycle has the following order: flowers, fruit, and seeds. In other words, seeds are the products of successful reproduction. The colors and scents of flowers serve to attract pollinators. Flowers and other plants can also be pollinated by wind. When a pollen grain meets the ovule and is successfully fertilized, the ovule develops into a seed. A seed consists of three parts: the embryo, the endosperm, and a seed coat. The embryo is a small plant that has started to develop, but this development is paused. Germination is when the embryo starts to grow again. The endosperm consists of proteins, carbohydrates, or fats. It typically serves as a food source for the embryo. The seed coat provides protection from disease, insects, and water.

> **Review Video: Kingdom Plantae**
> Visit mometrix.com/academy and enter code: 710084

The animal kingdom is comprised of more than one million species in about 30 phyla (the plant kingdom sometimes uses the term division). There about 800,000 species of insects alone, representing half of all animal species. The characteristics that distinguish members of the animal kingdom from members of other kingdoms are that they are multicellular, are heterotrophic, reproduce sexually (there are some exceptions), have cells that do not contain cell walls or photosynthetic pigments, can move at some stage of life, and can rapidly respond to the environment as a result of specialized tissues like nerve and muscle. Heterotrophic refers to the method of getting energy by eating food that has energy releasing substances. Plants, on the other hand, are autotrophs, which mean they make their own energy. During reproduction, animals have a diploid embryo in the blastula stage. This structure is unique to animals. The blastula resembles a fluid-filled ball.

The animal kingdom includes about one million species. Metazoans are multicellular animals. Food is ingested and enters a mesoderm-lined coelom (body cavity). Phylum porifera and coelenterate are exceptions. The taxonomy of animals involves grouping them into phyla according to body symmetry and plan, as well as the presence of or lack of segmentation. The more complex phyla that have a coelom and a digestive system are further classified as protostomes or deuterostomes according to blastula development. In protostomes, the blastula's blastopore (opening) forms a mouth. In deuterostomes, the blastopore forms an anus. Taxonomy schemes vary, but there are about 36 phyla of animals. The corresponding term for plants at this level is division. The most notable phyla include chordata, mollusca, porifera, cnidaria, platyhelminthes, nematoda, annelida, arthropoda, and echinodermata, which account for about 96 percent of all animal species.

> **Review Video: Kingdom Animalia**
> Visit mometrix.com/academy and enter code: 558413

These four animal phyla lack a coelom or have a pseudocoelom.

Porifera: These are sponges. They lack a coelom and get food as water flows through them. They are usually found in marine and sometimes in freshwater environments. They are perforated and diploblastic, meaning there are two layers of cells.

Cnidaria: Members of this phylum are hydrozoa, jellyfish, and obelia. They have radial symmetry, sac-like bodies, and a polyp or medusa (jellyfish) body plan. They are diploblastic, possessing both an ectoderm and an endoderm. Food can get in through a cavity, but members of this phylum do not have an anus.

Platyhelminthes: These are also known as flatworms. Classes include turbellaria (planarian) and trematoda (which include lung, liver, and blood fluke parasites). They have organs and bilateral symmetry. They have three layers of tissue: an ectoderm, a mesoderm, and an endoderm.

Nematoda: These are roundworms. Hookworms and many other parasites are members of this phylum. They have a pseudocoelom, which means the coelom is not completely enclosed within the mesoderm. They also have a digestive tract that runs directly from the mouth to the anus. They are nonsegmented.

Members of the protostomic phyla have mouths that are formed from blastopores.

Mollusca: Classes include bivalvia (organisms with two shells, such as clams, mussels, and oysters), gastropoda (snails and slugs), cephalopoda (octopus, squid, and chambered nautilus), scaphopoda, amphineura (chitons), and monoplacophora.

Annelida: This phylum includes the classes oligochaeta (earthworms), polychaeta (clam worms), and hirudinea (leeches). They have true coeloms enclosed within the mesoderm. They are segmented, have repeating units, and have a nerve trunk.

Arthropoda: The phylum is diverse and populous. Members can be found in all types of environments. They have external skeletons, jointed appendages, bilateral symmetry, and nerve cords. They also have open circulatory systems and sense organs. Subphyla include crustacea (lobster, barnacles, pill bugs, and daphnia), hexapoda (all insects, which have three body segments, six legs, and usual wings), myriapoda (centipedes and millipedes), and chelicerata (the horseshoe crab and arachnids). Pill bugs have gills. Bees, ants, and wasps belong to the order hymenoptera. Like several other insect orders, they undergo complete metamorphosis.

Members of the deuterostomic phyla have anuses that are formed from blastopores.

Echinodermata: Members of this phylum have radial symmetry, are marine organisms, and have a water vascular system. Classes include echinoidea (sea urchins and sand dollars), crinoidea (sea lilies), asteroidea (starfish), ophiuroidea (brittle stars), and holothuroidea (sea cucumbers).

Chordata: This phylum includes humans and all other vertebrates, as well as a few invertebrates (urochordata and cephalochordata). Members of this phylum include agnatha (lampreys and hagfish), gnathostomata, chondrichthyes (cartilaginous fish-like sharks, skates, and rays), osteichthyes (bony fishes, including ray-finned fish that humans eat), amphibians (frogs, salamander, and newts), reptiles (lizards, snakes, crocodiles, and dinosaurs), birds, and mammals.

Anatomy

Extrinsic refers to homeostatic systems that are controlled from outside the body. In higher animals, the nervous system and endocrine system help regulate body functions by responding to stimuli. Hormones in animals regulate many processes, including growth, metabolism, reproduction, and fluid balance. The names of hormones tend to end in "-one." Endocrine hormones are proteins or steroids. Steroid hormones (anabolic steroids) help control the manufacture of protein in muscles and bones.

Invertebrates do not have a backbone, whereas vertebrates do. The great majority of animal species (an estimated 98 percent) are invertebrates, including worms, jellyfish, mollusks, slugs, insects, and spiders. They comprise 30 phyla in all. Vertebrates belong to the phylum chordata. The vertebrate body has two cavities. The thoracic cavity holds the heart and lungs and the abdominal cavity holds the digestive organs. Animals with exoskeletons have skeletons on the outside. Examples are crabs and turtles. Animals with endoskeletons have skeletons on the inside. Examples are humans, tigers, birds, and reptiles.

The 11 major organ systems are: skeletal, muscular, nervous, digestive, respiratory, circulatory, skin, excretory, immune, endocrine, and reproductive.

Skeletal: This consists of the bones and joints. The skeletal system provides support for the body through its rigid structure, provides protection for internal organs, and works to make organisms motile. Growth hormone affects the rate of reproduction and the size of body cells, and also helps amino acids move through membranes.

Muscular: This includes the muscles. The muscular system allows the body to move and respond to its environment.

Nervous: This includes the brain, spinal cord, and nerves. The nervous system is a signaling system for intrabody communications among systems, responses to stimuli, and interaction within an environment. Signals are electrochemical. Conscious thoughts and memories and sense interpretation occur in the nervous system. It also controls involuntary muscles and functions, such as breathing and the beating of the heart.

> **Review Video: The Nervous System**
> Visit mometrix.com/academy and enter code: 708428

Digestive: This includes the mouth, pharynx, esophagus, stomach, intestines, rectum, anal canal, teeth, salivary glands, tongue, liver, gallbladder, pancreas, and appendix. The system helps change food into a form that the body can process and use for energy and nutrients. Food is eventually eliminated as solid waste. Digestive processes can be mechanical, such as chewing food and churning it in the stomach, and chemical, such as secreting hydrochloric acid to kill bacteria and converting protein to amino acids. The overall system converts large food particles into molecules so the body can use them. The small intestine transports the molecules to the circulatory system. The large intestine absorbs nutrients and prepares the unused portions of food for elimination.

Carbohydrates are the primary source of energy as they can be easily converted to glucose. Fats (oils or lipids) are usually not very water soluble, and vitamins A, D, E, and K are fat soluble. Fats are needed to help process these vitamins and can also store energy. Fats have the highest calorie value per gram (9,000 calories). Dietary fiber, or roughage, helps the excretory system. In humans, fiber can help regulate blood sugar levels, reduce heart disease, help food pass through the digestive system, and add bulk. Dietary minerals are chemical elements that are involved with biochemical functions in the body. Proteins consist of amino acids. Proteins are broken down in the body into amino acids that are used for protein biosynthesis or fuel. Vitamins are compounds that are not made by the body, but obtained through the diet. Water is necessary to prevent dehydration since water is lost through the excretory system and perspiration.

Respiratory: This includes the nose, pharynx, larynx, trachea, bronchi, and lungs. It is involved in gas exchange, which occurs in the alveoli. Fish have gills instead of lungs.

Circulatory: This includes the heart, blood, and blood vessels, such as veins, arteries, and capillaries. Blood transports oxygen and nutrients to cells and carbon dioxide to the lungs.

> **Review Video: Functions of the Circulatory System**
> Visit mometrix.com/academy and enter code: 376581

Skin (integumentary): This includes skin, hair, nails, sense receptors, sweat glands, and oil glands. The skin is a sense organ, provides an exterior barrier against disease, regulates body temperature through perspiration, manufactures chemicals and hormones, and provides a place for nerves from the nervous system and parts of the circulation system to travel through. Skin has three layers: epidermis, dermis, and subcutaneous. The epidermis is the thin, outermost, waterproof layer. Basal cells are located in the epidermis. The dermis contains the sweat glands, oil glands, and hair follicles. The subcutaneous layer has connective tissue, and also contains adipose (fat) tissue, nerves, arteries, and veins.

> **Review Video: Functions of the Integumentary System**
> Visit mometrix.com/academy and enter code: 398674

Excretory: This includes the kidneys, ureters, bladder, and urethra. The excretory system helps maintain the amount of fluids in the body. Wastes from the blood system and excess water are removed in urine. The system also helps remove solid waste.

Immune: This includes the lymphatic system, lymph nodes, lymph vessels, thymus, and spleen. Lymph fluid is moved throughout the body by lymph vessels that provide protection against disease. This system protects the body from external intrusions, such as microscopic organisms and foreign substances. It can also protect against some cancerous cells.

Endocrine: This includes the pituitary gland, pineal gland, hypothalamus, thyroid gland, parathyroids, thymus, adrenals, pancreas, ovaries, and testes. It controls systems and processes by secreting hormones into the blood system. Exocrine glands are those that secrete fluid into ducts. Endocrine glands secrete hormones directly into the blood stream without the use of ducts. Prostaglandin (tissue hormones) diffuses only a short distance from the tissue that created it, and influences nearby cells only. Adrenal glands are located above each kidney. The cortex secretes some sex hormones, as well as mineralocorticoids and glucocorticoids involved in immune suppression and stress response. The medulla secretes epinephrine and norepinephrine. Both elevate blood sugar, increase blood pressure, and accelerate heart rate. Epinephrine also stimulates heart muscle. The islets of Langerhans are clumped within the pancreas and secrete glucagon and insulin, thereby regulating blood sugar levels. The four parathyroid glands at the rear of the thyroid secrete parathyroid hormone.

Reproductive: In the male, this system includes the testes, vas deferens, urethra, prostate, penis, and scrotum. In the female, this system includes the ovaries, fallopian tubes (oviduct and uterine tubes), cervix, uterus, vagina, vulva, and mammary glands. Sexual reproduction helps provide genetic diversity as gametes from each parent contribute half the DNA to the zygote offspring. The system provides a method of transporting the male gametes to the female. It also allows for the growth and development of the embryo. Hormones involved are testosterone, interstitial cell stimulating hormone (ICSH), luteinizing hormone (LH), follicle stimulating hormone (FSH), and estrogen. Estrogens secreted from the ovaries include estradiol, estrone, and estriol. They encourage growth, among other things. Progesterone helps prepare the endometrium for pregnancy.

Based on whether or not and when an organism uses meiosis or mitosis, the three possible cycles of reproduction are haplontic, diplontic, and haplodiplontic. Fungi, green algae, and protozoa are haplontic. Animals and some brown algae and fungi are diplontic. Plants and some fungi are haplodiplontic. Diplontic organisms, like multicelled animals, have a dominant diploid life cycle. The haploid generation is simply the egg and sperm. Monoecious species are bisexual (hermaphroditic).

In this case, the individual has both male and female organs: sperm-bearing testicles and egg-bearing ovaries. Hermaphroditic species can self fertilize. Some worms are hermaphroditic. Cross fertilization is when individuals exchange genetic information. Most animal species are dioecious, meaning individuals are distinctly male or female.

Biological Relationships

As heterotrophs, animals can be further classified as carnivores, herbivores, omnivores, and parasites. Predation refers to a predator that feeds on another organism, which results in its death. Detritivory refers to heterotrophs that consume organic dead matter. Carnivores are animals that are meat eaters. Herbivores are plant eaters, and omnivores eat both meat and plants. A parasite's food source is its host. A parasite lives off of a host, which does not benefit from the interaction. Nutrients can be classified as carbohydrates, fats, fiber, minerals, proteins, vitamins, and water. Each supply a specific substance required for various species to survive, grow, and reproduce. A calorie is a measurement of heat energy. It can be used to represent both how much energy a food can provide and how much energy an organism needs to live. Biochemical cycles are how chemical elements required by living organisms cycle between living and nonliving organisms. Elements that are frequently required are phosphorus, sulfur, oxygen, carbon, gaseous nitrogen, and water. Elements can go through gas cycles, sedimentary cycles, or both. Elements circulate through the air in a gas cycle and from land to water in a sedimentary one.

A food chain is a linking of organisms in a community that is based on how they use each other as food sources. Each link in the chain consumes the link above it and is consumed by the link below it. The exceptions are the organism at the top of the food chain and the organism at the bottom.

Biomagnification (bioamplification): This refers to an increase in concentration of a substance within a food chain. Examples are pesticides or mercury. Mercury is emitted from coal-fired power plants and gets into the water supply, where it is eaten by a fish. A larger fish eats smaller fish, and humans eat fish. The concentration of mercury in humans has now risen. Biomagnification is affected by the persistence of a chemical, whether it can be broken down and negated, food chain energetics, and whether organisms can reduce or negate the substance.

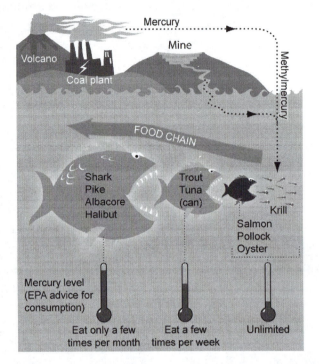

A food web consists of interconnected food chains in a community. The organisms can be linked to show the direction of energy flow. Energy flow in this sense is used to refer to the actual caloric flow through a system from trophic level to trophic level. Trophic level refers to a link in a food chain or a level of nutrition. The 10% rule is that from trophic level to level, about 90% of the energy is lost (in the form of heat, for example). The lowest trophic level consists of primary producers (usually plants), then primary consumers, then secondary consumers, and finally tertiary consumers (large carnivores). The final link is decomposers, which break down the consumers at the top. Food chains usually do not contain more than six links. These links may also be referred to as ecological pyramids.

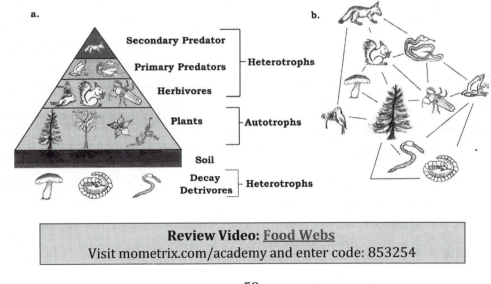

Review Video: Food Webs
Visit mometrix.com/academy and enter code: 853254

- 58 -

Ecosystem stability is a concept that states that a stable ecosystem is perfectly efficient. Seasonal changes or expected climate fluctuations are balanced by homeostasis. It also states that interspecies interactions are part of the balance of the system. Four principles of ecosystem stability are that waste disposal and nutrient replenishment by recycling is complete, the system uses sunlight as an energy source, biodiversity remains, and populations are stable in that they do not over consume resources. Ecologic succession is the concept that states that there is an orderly progression of change within a community. An example of primary succession is that over hundreds of years bare rock decomposes to sand, which eventually leads to soil formation, which eventually leads to the growth of grasses and trees. Secondary succession occurs after a disturbance or major event that greatly affects a community, such as a wild fire or construction of a dam.

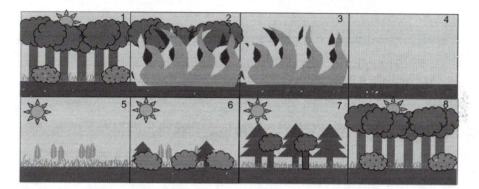

Population is a measure of how many individuals exist in a specific area. It can be used to measure the size of human, plant, or animal groups. Population growth depends on many factors. Factors that can limit the number of individuals in a population include lack of resources such as food and water, space, habitat destruction, competition, disease, and predators. Exponential growth refers to an unlimited rising growth rate. This kind of growth can be plotted on a chart in the shape of a J. Carrying capacity is the population size that can be sustained. The world's population is about 6.8 billion and growing. The human population has not yet reached its carrying capacity. Population dynamics refers to how a population changes over time and the factors that cause changes. An S-shaped curve shows that population growth has leveled off. Biotic potential refers to the maximum reproductive capacity of a population given ideal environmental conditions.

Biological concepts:

Territoriality: This refers to members of a species protecting areas from other members of their species and from other species. Species members claim specific areas as their own.

Dominance: This refers to the species in a community that is the most populous.

Altruism: This is when a species or individual in a community exhibits behaviors that benefit another individual at a cost to itself. In biology, altruism does not have to be a conscious sacrifice.

Threat display: This refers to behavior by an organism that is intended to intimidate or frighten away members of its own or another species.

The principle of **competitive exclusion** (Gause's Law) states that if there are limited or insufficient resources and species are competing for them, these species will not be able to co-exist. The result is that one of the species will become extinct or be forced to undergo a behavioral or evolutionary change. Another way to say this is that "complete competitors cannot coexist."

A **community** is any number of species interacting within a given area. A **niche** is the role of a species within a community. **Species diversity** refers to the number of species within a community and their populations. A **biome** refers to an area in which species are associated because of climate. The six major biomes in North America are desert, tropical rain forest, grassland, coniferous forest, deciduous forest, and tundra.

Biotic: Biotic factors are the living factors, such as other organisms, that affect a community or population. Abiotic factors are nonliving factors that affect a community or population, such as facets of the environment.

Ecology: Ecology is the study of plants, animals, their environments, and how they interact.

Ecosystem: An ecosystem is a community of species and all of the environment factors that affect them.

Biomass: In ecology, biomass refers to the mass of one or all of the species (species biomass) in an ecosystem or area.

Predation, parasitism, commensalism, and mutualism are all types of species interactions that affect species populations. **Intraspecific relationships** are relationships among members of a species. **Interspecific relationships** are relationships between members of different species.

Predation: This is a relationship in which one individual feeds on another (the prey), causing the prey to die. **Mimicry** is an adaptation developed as a response to predation. It refers to an organism that has a similar appearance to another species, which is meant to fool the predator into thinking the organism is more dangerous than it really is. Two examples are the drone fly and the io moth. The fly looks like a bee, but cannot sting. The io moth has markings on its wings that make it look like an owl. The moth can startle predators and gain time to escape. Predators can also use mimicry to lure their prey.

Commensalism: This refers to interspecific relationships in which one of the organisms benefits.

Mutualism, competition, and parasitism are all types of commensalism.

Mutualism: This is a relationship in which both organisms benefit from an interaction.

Competition: This is a relationship in which both organisms are harmed.

Parasitism: This is a relationship in which one organism benefits and the other is harmed.

> **Review Video: Mutualism, Commensalism, and Parasitism**
> Visit mometrix.com/academy and enter code: 757249

Chemistry

Atoms

Matter refers to substances that have mass and occupy space (or volume). The traditional definition of matter describes it as having three states: solid, liquid, and gas. These different states are caused by differences in the distances and angles between molecules or atoms, which result in differences in the energy that binds them. Solid structures are rigid or nearly rigid and have strong bonds. Molecules or atoms of liquids move around and have weak bonds, although they are not weak enough to readily break. Molecules or atoms of gases move almost independently of each other, are typically far apart, and do not form bonds. The current definition of matter describes it as having four states. The fourth is plasma, which is an ionized gas that has some electrons that are described as free because they are not bound to an atom or molecule.

All matter consists of atoms. Atoms consist of a nucleus and electrons. The nucleus consists of protons and neutrons. The properties of these are measurable; they have mass and an electrical charge. The nucleus is positively charged due to the presence of protons. Electrons are negatively charged and orbit the nucleus. The nucleus has considerably more mass than the surrounding electrons. Atoms can bond together to make molecules. Atoms that have an equal number of protons and electrons are electrically neutral. If the number of protons and electrons in an atom is not equal, the atom has a positive or negative charge and is an ion.

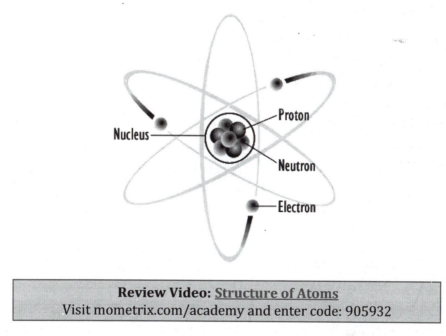

Review Video: Structure of Atoms
Visit mometrix.com/academy and enter code: 905932

An element is matter with one particular type of atom. It can be identified by its atomic number, or the number of protons in its nucleus. There are approximately 117 elements currently known, 94 of which occur naturally on Earth. Elements from the periodic table include hydrogen, carbon, iron, helium, mercury, and oxygen. Atoms combine to form molecules. For example, two atoms of hydrogen (H) and one atom of oxygen (O) combine to form water (H_2O).

Compounds are substances containing two or more elements. Compounds are formed by chemical reactions and frequently have different properties than the original elements. Compounds are decomposed by a chemical reaction rather than separated by a physical one. Solutions are homogeneous mixtures composed of two or more substances that have become one. Mixtures contain two or more substances that are combined but have not reacted chemically with each other. Mixtures can be separated using physical methods, while compounds cannot.

A solution is a homogeneous mixture. A mixture is two or more different substances that are mixed together, but not combined chemically. Homogeneous mixtures are those that are uniform in their composition. Solutions consist of a solute (the substance that is dissolved) and a solvent (the substance that does the dissolving). An example is sugar water. The solvent is the water and the solute is the sugar. The intermolecular attraction between the solvent and the solute is called solvation. Hydration refers to solutions in which water is the solvent. Solutions are formed when the forces of the molecules of the solute and the solvent are as strong as the individual molecular forces of the solute and the solvent. An example is that salt (NaCl) dissolves in water to create a solution. The Na^+ and the Cl^- ions in salt interact with the molecules of water and vice versa to overcome the individual molecular forces of the solute and the solvent.

Elements are represented in upper case letters. If there is no subscript, it indicates there is only one atom of the element. Otherwise, the subscript indicates the number of atoms. In molecular formulas, elements are organized according to the Hill system. Carbon is first, hydrogen comes next, and the remaining elements are listed in alphabetical order. If there is no carbon, all elements are listed alphabetically. There are a couple of exceptions to these rules. First, oxygen is usually listed last in oxides. Second, in ionic compounds the positive ion is listed first, followed by the negative ion. In CO_2, for example, C indicates 1 atom of carbon and O_2 indicates 2 atoms of oxygen. The compound is carbon dioxide. The formula for ammonia (an ionic compound) is NH_3, which is one atom of nitrogen and three of hydrogen. H_2O is two atoms of hydrogen and one of oxygen. Sugar is $C_6H_{12}O_6$, which is 6 atoms of carbon, 12 of hydrogen, and 6 of oxygen.

An **atom** is one of the most basic units of matter. An atom consists of a central nucleus surrounded by electrons. The **nucleus** of an atom consists of protons and neutrons. It is positively charged, dense, and heavier than the surrounding electrons. The plural form of nucleus is nuclei. **Neutrons** are the uncharged atomic particles contained within the nucleus. The number of neutrons in a nucleus can be represented as "N." Along with neutrons, **protons** make up the nucleus of an atom. The number of protons in the nucleus determines the atomic number of an element. Carbon atoms, for example, have six protons. The atomic number of carbon is 6. **Nucleon** refers collectively to neutrons and protons. **Electrons** are atomic particles that are negatively charged and orbit the nucleus of an atom. The number of protons minus the number of electrons indicates the charge of an atom.

The **atomic number** of an element refers to the number of protons in the nucleus of an atom. It is a unique identifier. It can be represented as Z. Atoms with a neutral charge have an atomic number that is equal to the number of electrons. **Atomic mass** is also known as the mass number. The atomic mass is the total number of protons and neutrons in the nucleus of an atom. It is referred to as "A." The atomic mass (A) is equal to the number of protons (Z) plus the number of neutrons (N).

- 62 -

This can be represented by the equation A = Z + N. The mass of electrons in an atom is basically insignificant because it is so small. **Atomic weight** may sometimes be referred to as "relative atomic mass," but should not be confused with atomic mass. Atomic weight is the ratio of the average mass per atom of a sample (which can include various isotopes of an element) to 1/12 of the mass of an atom of carbon-12.

Chemical properties are qualities of a substance which can't be determined by simply looking at the substance and must be determined through chemical reactions. Some chemical properties of elements include: atomic number, electron configuration, electrons per shell, electronegativity, atomic radius, and isotopes.

In contrast to chemical properties, **physical properties** can be observed or measured without chemical reactions. These include properties such as color, elasticity, mass, volume, and temperature. **Mass** is a measure of the amount of substance in an object. **Weight** is a measure of the gravitational pull of Earth on an object. **Volume** is a measure of the amount of space occupied. There are many formulas to determine volume. For example, the volume of a cube is the length of one side cubed (a^3) and the volume of a rectangular prism is length times width times height ($l \cdot w \cdot h$). The volume of an irregular shape can be determined by how much water it displaces. **Density** is a measure of the amount of mass per unit volume. The formula to find density is mass divided by volume ($D=m/V$). It is expressed in terms of mass per cubic unit, such as grams per cubic centimeter (g/cm^3). **Specific gravity** is a measure of the ratio of a substance's density compared to the density of water.

> **Review Video: Mass, Weight, Volume, Density, and Specific Gravity**
> Visit mometrix.com/academy and enter code: 920570

Both physical changes and chemical reactions are everyday occurrences. Physical changes do not result in different substances. For example, when water becomes ice it has undergone a physical change, but not a chemical change. It has changed its form, but not its composition. It is still H_2O. Chemical properties are concerned with the constituent particles that make up the physicality of a substance. Chemical properties are apparent when chemical changes occur. The chemical properties of a substance are influenced by its electron configuration, which is determined in part by the number of protons in the nucleus (the atomic number). Carbon, for example, has 6 protons and 6 electrons. It is an element's outermost valence electrons that mainly determine its chemical properties. Chemical reactions may release or consume energy.

Periodic Table

The periodic table groups elements with similar chemical properties together. The grouping of elements is based on atomic structure. It shows periodic trends of physical and chemical properties and identifies families of elements with similar properties. It is a common model for organizing and understanding elements. In the periodic table, each element has its own cell that includes varying amounts of information presented in symbol form about the properties of the element. Cells in the table are arranged in rows (periods) and columns (groups or families). At minimum, a cell includes the symbol for the element and its atomic number. The cell for hydrogen, for example, which appears first in the upper left corner, includes an "H" and a "1" above the letter. Elements are ordered by atomic number, left to right, top to bottom.

In the periodic table, the groups are the columns numbered 1 through 18 that group elements with similar outer electron shell configurations. Since the configuration of the outer electron shell is one of the primary factors affecting an element's chemical properties, elements within the same group have similar chemical properties. Previous naming conventions for groups have included the use of Roman numerals and upper-case letters. Currently, the periodic table groups are: Group 1, alkali metals; Group 2, alkaline earth metals; Groups 3-12, transition metals; Group 13, boron family; Group 14; carbon family; Group 15, pnictogens; Group 16, chalcogens; Group 17, halogens; Group 18, noble gases.

In the periodic table, there are seven periods (rows), and within each period there are blocks that group elements with the same outer electron subshell (more on this in the next section). The number of electrons in that outer shell determines which group an element belongs to within a given block. Each row's number (1, 2, 3, etc.) corresponds to the highest number electron shell that is in use. For example, row 2 uses only electron shells 1 and 2, while row 7 uses all shells from 1-7.

Atomic radii will decrease from left to right across a period (row) on the periodic table. In a group (column), there is an increase in the atomic radii of elements from top to bottom. Ionic radii will be smaller than the atomic radii for metals, but the opposite is true for non-metals. From left to right, electronegativity, or an atom's likeliness of taking another atom's electrons, increases. In a group, electronegativity decreases from top to bottom. Ionization energy or the amount of energy needed to get rid of an atom's outermost electron, increases across a period and decreases down a group. Electron affinity will become more negative across a period but will not change much within a group. The melting point decreases from top to bottom in the metal groups and increases from top to bottom in the non-metal groups.

Group→1	2	3	4	5	6	7	8	9	10	11	12	13	14	15	16	17	18
↓Period																	
1 H																	2 He
3 Li	4 Be											5 B	6 C	7 N	8 O	9 F	10 Ne
11 Na	12 Mg											13 Al	14 Si	15 P	16 S	17 Cl	18 Ar
19 K	20 Ca	21 Sc	22 Ti	23 V	24 Cr	25 Mn	26 Fe	27 Co	28 Ni	29 Cu	30 Zn	31 Ga	32 Ge	33 As	34 Se	35 Br	36 Kr
37 Rb	38 Sr	39 Y	40 Zr	41 Nb	42 Mo	43 Tc	44 Ru	45 Rh	46 Pd	47 Ag	48 Cd	49 In	50 Sn	51 Sb	52 Te	53 I	54 Xe
55 Cs	56 Ba	*	72 Hf	73 Ta	74 W	75 Re	76 Os	77 Ir	78 Pt	79 Au	80 Hg	81 Tl	82 Pb	83 Bi	84 Po	85 At	86 Rn
87 Fr	88 Ra	**	104 Rf	105 Db	106 Sg	107 Bh	108 Hs	109 Mt	110 Ds	111 Rg	112 Cn	113 Uut	114 Fl	115 Uup	116 Lv	117 Uus	118 Uuo

*	57 La	58 Ce	59 Pr	60 Nd	61 Pm	62 Sm	63 Eu	64 Gd	65 Tb	66 Dy	67 Ho	68 Er	69 Tm	70 Yb	71 Lu
**	89 Ac	90 Th	91 Pa	92 U	93 Np	94 Pu	95 Am	96 Cm	97 Bk	98 Cf	99 Es	100 Fm	101 Md	102 No	103 Lr

Electrons

Electrons are subatomic particles that orbit the nucleus at various levels commonly referred to as layers, shells, or clouds. The orbiting electron or electrons account for only a fraction of the atom's mass. They are much smaller than the nucleus, are negatively charged, and exhibit wave-like characteristics. Electrons are part of the lepton family of elementary particles. Electrons can occupy orbits that are varying distances away from the nucleus, and tend to occupy the lowest energy level they can. If an atom has all its electrons in the lowest available positions, it has a stable electron arrangement. The outermost electron shell of an atom in its uncombined state is known as the valence shell. The electrons there are called valence electrons, and it is their number that determines bonding behavior. Atoms tend to react in a manner that will allow them to fill or empty their valence shells.

There are seven electron shells. One is closest to the nucleus and seven is the farthest away. Electron shells can also be identified with the letters K, L, M, N, O, P, and Q. Traditionally, there were four subshells identified by the first letter of their descriptive name: s (sharp), p (principal), d (diffuse), and f (fundamental). The maximum number of electrons for each subshell is as follows: s is 2, p is 6, d is 10, and f is 14. Every shell has an s subshell, the second shell and those above also have a p subshell, the third shell and those above also have a d subshell, and so on. Each subshell contains atomic orbitals, which describes the wave-like characteristics of an electron or a pair of electrons expressed as two angles and the distance from the nucleus. Atomic orbital is a concept used to express the likelihood of an electron's position in accordance with the idea of wave-particle duality.

Electron configuration: This is a trend whereby electrons fill shells and subshells in an element in a particular order and with a particular number of electrons. The chemical properties of the elements reflect their electron configurations. Energy levels (shells) do not have to be completely filled before the next one begins to be filled. An example of electron configuration notation is $1s^22s^22p^5$, where the first number is the row (period), or shell. The letter refers to the subshell of the shell, and the number in superscript is the number of electrons in the subshell. A common shorthand method for electron configuration notation is to use a noble gas (in a bracket) to abbreviate the shells that elements have in common. For example, the electron configuration for neon is $1s^22s^22p^6$. The configuration for phosphorus is $1s^22s^22p^63s^23p^3$, which can be written as $[Ne]3s^23p^3$. Subshells are filled in the following manner: 1s, 2s, 2p, 3s, 3p, 4s, 3d, 4p, 5s, 4d, 5p, 6s, 4f, 5d, 6p, 7s, 5f, 6d, and 7p.

Most atoms are neutral since the positive charge of the protons in the nucleus is balanced by the negative charge of the surrounding electrons. Electrons are transferred between atoms when they come into contact with each other. This creates a molecule or atom in which the number of electrons does not equal the number of protons, which gives it a positive or negative charge. A negative ion is created when an atom gains electrons, while a positive ion is created when an atom loses electrons. An ionic bond is formed between ions with opposite charges. The resulting compound is neutral. Ionization refers to the process by which neutral particles are ionized into charged particles. Gases and plasmas can be partially or fully ionized through ionization.

Atoms interact by transferring or sharing the electrons furthest from the nucleus. Known as the outer or valence electrons, they are responsible for the chemical properties of an element. Bonds between atoms are created when electrons are paired up by being transferred or shared. If electrons are transferred from one atom to another, the bond is ionic. If electrons are shared, the bond is covalent. Atoms of the same element may bond together to form molecules or crystalline solids. When two or more different types of atoms bind together chemically, a compound is made. The physical properties of compounds reflect the nature of the interactions among their molecules. These interactions are determined by the structure of the molecule, including the atoms they consist of and the distances and angles between them.

Isotopes and Molecules

The number of protons in an atom determines the element of that atom. For instance, all helium atoms have exactly two protons, and all oxygen atoms have exactly eight protons. If two atoms have the same number of protons, then they are the same element. However, the number of neutrons in two atoms can be different without the atoms being different elements. Isotope is the term used to distinguish between atoms that have the same number of protons but a different number of neutrons. The names of isotopes have the element name with the mass number. Recall that the mass number is the number of protons plus the number of neutrons. For example, carbon-12 refers to an atom that has 6 protons, which makes it carbon, and 6 neutrons. In other words, 6 protons + 6 neutrons = 12. Carbon-13 has six protons and seven neutrons, and carbon-14 has six protons and eight neutrons. Isotopes can also be written with the mass number in superscript before the element symbol. For example, carbon-12 can be written as ^{12}C.

The important properties of water (H_2O) are high polarity, hydrogen bonding, cohesiveness, adhesiveness, high specific heat, high latent heat, and high heat of vaporization. It is essential to life as we know it, as water is one of the main if not the main constituent of many living things. Water is a liquid at room temperature. The high specific heat of water means it resists the breaking of its hydrogen bonds and resists heat and motion, which is why it has a relatively high boiling point and high vaporization point. It also resists temperature change. Water is peculiar in that its solid state floats in its liquid state. Most substances are denser in their solid forms. Water is cohesive, which means it is attracted to itself. It is also adhesive, which means it readily attracts other molecules. If water tends to adhere to another substance, the substance is said to be hydrophilic. Water makes a good solvent. Substances, particularly those with polar ions and molecules, readily dissolve in water. Electrons in an atom can orbit different levels around the nucleus. They can absorb or release energy, which can change the location of their orbit or even allow them to break free from the atom. The outermost layer is the valence layer, which contains the valence electrons. The valence layer tends to have or share eight electrons. Molecules are formed by a chemical bond between atoms, a bond which occurs at the valence level.

Two basic types of bonds are covalent and ionic. A covalent bond is formed when atoms share electrons. An ionic bond is formed when an atom transfers an electron to another atom. A hydrogen bond is a weak bond between a hydrogen atom of one molecule and an electronegative atom (such as nitrogen, oxygen, or fluorine) of another molecule. The Van der Waals force is a weak force between molecules. This type of force is much weaker than actual chemical bonds between atoms.

Reactions

Chemical reactions measured in human time can take place quickly or slowly. They can take fractions of a second or billions of years. The rates of chemical reactions are determined by how frequently reacting atoms and molecules interact. Rates are also influenced by the temperature and various properties (such as shape) of the reacting materials. Catalysts accelerate chemical reactions, while inhibitors decrease reaction rates. Some types of reactions release energy in the form of heat and light. Some types of reactions involve the transfer of either electrons or hydrogen ions between reacting ions, molecules, or atoms. In other reactions, chemical bonds are broken down by heat or light to form reactive radicals with electrons that will readily form new bonds.

Processes such as the formation of ozone and greenhouse gases in the atmosphere and the burning and processing of fossil fuels are controlled by radical reactions.

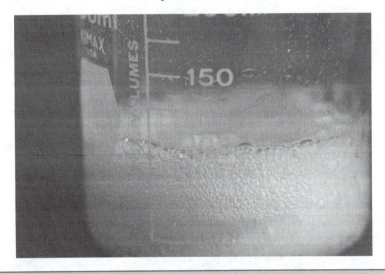

Review Video: Chemical Reactions
Visit mometrix.com/academy and enter code: 579876

Review Video: Catalysts
Visit mometrix.com/academy and enter code: 288189

Chemical equations describe chemical reactions. The reactants are on the left side before the arrow and the products are on the right side after the arrow. The arrow indicates the reaction or change. The coefficient, or stoichiometric coefficient, is the number before the element, and indicates the ratio of reactants to products in terms of moles. The equation for the formation of water from hydrogen and oxygen, for example, is $2H_{2(g)} + O_{2(g)} \rightarrow 2H_2O_{(l)}$. The 2 preceding hydrogen and water is the coefficient, which means there are 2 moles of hydrogen and 2 of water. There is 1 mole of oxygen, which does not have to be indicated with the number 1. In parentheses, g stands for gas, l stands for liquid, s stands for solid, and aq stands for aqueous solution (a substance dissolved in water). Charges are shown in superscript for individual ions, but not for ionic compounds. Polyatomic ions are separated by parentheses so the ion will not be confused with the number of ions.

Review Video: Balanced Chemical Equations
Visit mometrix.com/academy and enter code: 839820

An unbalanced equation is one that does not follow the law of conservation of mass, which states that matter can only be changed, not created. If an equation is unbalanced, the numbers of atoms indicated by the stoichiometric coefficients on each side of the arrow will not be equal. Start by writing the formulas for each species in the reaction. Count the atoms on each side and determine if the number is equal. Coefficients must be whole numbers. Fractional amounts, such as half a molecule, are not possible. Equations can be balanced by multiplying the coefficients by a constant that will produce the smallest possible whole number coefficient. $H_2 + O_2 \rightarrow H_2O$ is an example of an unbalanced equation. The balanced equation is $2H_2 + O_2 \rightarrow 2H_2O$, which indicates that it takes two moles of hydrogen and one of oxygen to produce two moles of water.

> **Review Video: How to Balance a Chemical Equation**
> Visit mometrix.com/academy and enter code: 341228

One way to organize chemical reactions is to sort them into two categories: oxidation/reduction reactions (also called redox reactions) and metathesis reactions (which include acid/base reactions). Oxidation/reduction reactions can involve the transfer of one or more electrons, or they can occur as a result of the transfer of oxygen, hydrogen, or halogen atoms. The species that loses electrons is oxidized and is referred to as the reducing agent. The species that gains electrons is reduced and is referred to as the oxidizing agent. The element undergoing oxidation experiences an increase in its oxidation number, while the element undergoing reduction experiences a decrease in its oxidation number. Single replacement reactions are types of oxidation/reduction reactions. In a single replacement reaction, electrons are transferred from one chemical species to another. The transfer of electrons results in changes in the nature and charge of the species.

> **Review Video: Reduction**
> Visit mometrix.com/academy and enter code: 317289

Single substitution, displacement, or replacement reactions are when one reactant is displaced by another to form the final product ($A + BC \rightarrow B + AC$). Single substitution reactions can be cationic or anionic. When a piece of copper (Cu) is placed into a solution of silver nitrate ($AgNO_3$), the solution turns blue. The copper appears to be replaced with a silvery-white material. The equation is $2AgNO_3 + Cu \rightarrow Cu(NO_3)2 + 2Ag$. When this reaction takes place, the copper dissolves and the silver in the silver nitrate solution precipitates (becomes a solid), thus resulting in copper nitrate and silver. Copper and silver have switched places in the nitrate.

Combination, or synthesis, reactions: In a combination reaction, two or more reactants combine to form a single product ($A + B \rightarrow C$). These reactions are also called synthesis or addition reactions. An example is burning hydrogen in air to produce water. The equation is $2H_{2\,(g)} + O_{2\,(g)} \rightarrow 2H_2O_{\,(l)}$. Another example is when water and sulfur trioxide react to form sulfuric acid. The equation is $H_2O + SO_3 \rightarrow H_2SO_4$.

Double displacement, double replacement, substitution, metathesis, or ion exchange reactions are when ions or bonds are exchanged by two compounds to form different compounds ($AC + BD \rightarrow AD + BC$). An example of this is that silver nitrate and sodium chloride form two different products (silver chloride and sodium nitrate) when they react. The formula for this reaction is $AgNO_3 + NaCl \rightarrow AgCl + NaNO_3$.

Double replacement reactions are metathesis reactions. In a double replacement reaction, the chemical reactants exchange ions but the oxidation state stays the same. One of the indicators of this is the formation of a solid precipitate. In acid/base reactions, an acid is a compound that can donate a proton, while a base is a compound that can accept a proton. In these types of reactions, the acid and base react to form a salt and water. When the proton is donated, the base becomes water and the remaining ions form a salt. One method of determining whether a reaction is an oxidation/reduction or a metathesis reaction is that the oxidation number of atoms does not change during a metathesis reaction.

A neutralization, acid-base, or proton transfer reaction is when one compound acquires H+ from another. These types of reactions are also usually double displacement reactions. The acid has an H+ that is transferred to the base and neutralized to form a salt.

Decomposition (or desynthesis, decombination, or deconstruction) reactions; in a decomposition reaction, a reactant is broken down into two or more products (A → B + C). These reactions are also called analysis reactions. Thermal decomposition is caused by heat. Electrolytic decomposition is due to electricity. An example of this type of reaction is the decomposition of water into hydrogen and oxygen gas. The equation is $2H_2O \rightarrow 2H_2 + O_2$. Decomposition is considered a chemical reaction whereby a single compound breaks down into component parts or simpler compounds. When a compound or substance separates into these simpler substances, the byproducts are often substances that are different from the original. Decomposition can be viewed as the opposite of combination reactions. Most decomposition reactions are endothermic. Heat needs to be added for the chemical reaction to occur. Separation processes can be mechanical or chemical, and usually involve re-organizing a mixture of substances without changing their chemical nature. The separated products may differ from the original mixture in terms of chemical or physical properties. Types of separation processes include filtration, crystallization, distillation, and chromatography. Basically, decomposition breaks down one compound into two or more compounds or substances that are different from the original; separation sorts the substances from the original mixture into like substances.

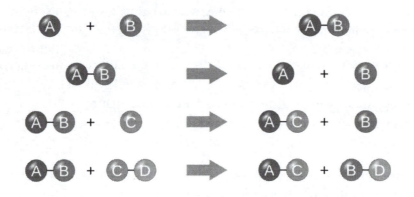

Endothermic reactions are chemical reactions that absorb heat and exothermic reactions are chemical reactions that release heat. Reactants are the substances that are consumed during a reaction, while products are the substances that are produced or formed. A balanced equation is one that uses reactants, products, and coefficients in such a way that the number of each type of atom (law of conservation of mass) and the total charge remains the same. The reactants are on the left side of the arrow and the products are on the right. The heat difference between endothermic and exothermic reactions is caused by bonds forming and breaking. If more energy is needed to break the reactant bonds than is released when they form, the reaction is endothermic. Heat is absorbed and the environmental temperature decreases. If more energy is released when product

- 70 -

bonds form than is needed to break the reactant bonds, the reaction is exothermic. Heat is released and the environmental temperature increases.

The collision theory states that for a chemical reaction to occur, atoms or molecules have to collide with each other with a certain amount of energy. A certain amount of energy is required to breach the activation barrier. Heating a mixture will raise the energy levels of the molecules and the rate of reaction (the time it takes for a reaction to complete). Generally, the rate of reaction is doubled for every 10 degrees Celsius temperature increase. However, the increase needed to double a reaction rate increases as the temperature climbs. This is due to the increase in collision frequency that occurs as the temperature increases. Other factors that can affect the rate of reaction are surface area, concentration, pressure, and the presence of a catalyst.

The particles of an atom's nucleus (the protons and neutrons) are bound together by nuclear force, also known as residual strong force. Unlike chemical reactions, which involve electrons, nuclear reactions occur when two nuclei or nuclear particles collide. This results in the release or absorption of energy and products that are different from the initial particles. The energy released in a nuclear reaction can take various forms, including the release of kinetic energy of the product particles and the emission of very high energy photons known as gamma rays. Some energy may also remain in the nucleus. Radioactivity refers to the particles emitted from nuclei as a result of nuclear instability. There are many nuclear isotopes that are unstable and can spontaneously emit some kind of radiation. The most common types of radiation are alpha, beta, and gamma radiation, but there are several other varieties of radioactive decay.

Inorganic and Organic

The terms inorganic and organic have become less useful over time as their definitions have changed. Historically, inorganic molecules were defined as those of a mineral nature that were not created by biological processes. Organic molecules were defined as those that were produced biologically by a "life process" or "vital force." It was then discovered that organic compounds could be synthesized without a life process.

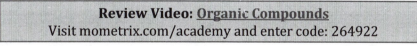
Review Video: Organic Compounds
Visit mometrix.com/academy and enter code: 264922

Currently, molecules containing carbon are considered organic. Carbon is largely responsible for creating biological diversity, and is more capable than all other elements of forming large, complex, and diverse molecules of an organic nature. Carbon often completes its valence shell by sharing electrons with other atoms in four covalent bonds, which is also known as tetravalence.

The main trait of inorganic compounds is that they lack carbon. Inorganic compounds include mineral salts, metals and alloys, non-metallic compounds such as phosphorus, and metal complexes. A metal complex has a central atom (or ion) bonded to surrounding ligands (molecules or anions). The ligands sacrifice the donor atoms (in the form of at least one pair of electrons) to the central atom. Many inorganic compounds are ionic, meaning they form ionic bonds rather than share electrons. They may have high melting points because of this. They may also be colorful, but this is not an absolute identifier of an inorganic compound. Salts, which are inorganic compounds, are an example of inorganic bonding of cations and anions. Some examples of salts are magnesium chloride ($MgCl_2$) and sodium oxide (Na_2O). Oxides, carbonates, sulfates, and halides are classes of inorganic compounds. They are typically poor conductors, are very water soluble, and crystallize easily. Minerals and silicates are also inorganic compounds.

Two of the main characteristics of organic compounds are that they include carbon and are formed by covalent bonds. Carbon can form long chains, double and triple bonds, and rings. While inorganic compounds tend to have high melting points, organic compounds tend to melt at temperatures below 300° C. They also tend to boil, sublimate, and decompose below this temperature. Unlike inorganic compounds, they are not very water soluble. Organic molecules are organized into functional groups based on their specific atoms, which helps determine how they will react chemically. A few groups are alkanes, nitro, alkenes, sulfides, amines, and carbolic acids. The hydroxyl group (-OH) consists of alcohols. These molecules are polar, which increases their solubility. By some estimates, there are more than 16 million organic compounds.

Nomenclature refers to the manner in which a compound is named. First, it must be determined whether the compound is ionic (formed through electron transfer between cations and anions) or molecular (formed through electron sharing between molecules). When dealing with an ionic compound, the name is determined using the standard naming conventions for ionic compounds. This involves indicating the positive element first (the charge must be defined when there is more than one option for the valency) followed by the negative element plus the appropriate suffix. The rules for naming a molecular compound are as follows: write elements in order of increasing group number and determine the prefix by determining the number of atoms. Exclude mono for the first atom. The name for CO_2, for example, is carbon dioxide. The end of oxygen is dropped and "ide" is added to make oxide, and the prefix "di" is used to indicate there are two atoms of oxygen.

Acids and Bases

The potential of hydrogen (pH) is a measurement of the concentration of hydrogen ions in a substance in terms of the number of moles of H^+ per liter of solution. All substances fall between 0 and 14 on the pH scale. A lower pH indicates a higher H^+ concentration, while a higher pH indicates a lower H^+ concentration. Pure water has a neutral pH, which is 7. Anything with a pH lower than water (0-7) is considered acidic. Anything with a pH higher than water (7-14) is a base. Drain cleaner, soap, baking soda, ammonia, egg whites, and sea water are common bases. Urine, stomach acid, citric acid, vinegar, hydrochloric acid, and battery acid are acids. A pH indicator is a substance that acts as a detector of hydrogen or hydronium ions. It is halochromic, meaning it changes color to indicate that hydrogen or hydronium ions have been detected.

When they are dissolved in aqueous solutions, some properties of acids are that they conduct electricity, change blue litmus paper to red, have a sour taste, react with bases to neutralize them, and react with active metals to free hydrogen. A weak acid is one that does not donate all of its protons or disassociate completely. Strong acids include hydrochloric, hydriodic, hydrobromic, perchloric, nitric, and sulfuric. They ionize completely. Superacids are those that are stronger than 100 percent sulfuric acid. They include fluoroantimonic, magic, and perchloric acids. Acids can be used in pickling, a process used to remove rust and corrosion from metals. They are also used as catalysts in the processing of minerals and the production of salts and fertilizers. Phosphoric acid (H_3PO_4) is added to sodas and other acids are added to foods as preservatives or to add taste.

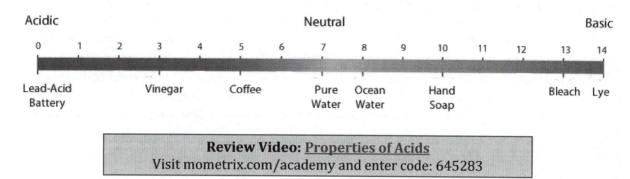

Review Video: **Properties of Acids**
Visit mometrix.com/academy and enter code: 645283

When they are dissolved in aqueous solutions, some properties of bases are that they conduct electricity, change red litmus paper to blue, feel slippery, and react with acids to neutralize their properties. A weak base is one that does not completely ionize in an aqueous solution, and usually has a low pH. Strong bases can free protons in very weak acids. Examples of strong bases are hydroxide compounds such as potassium, barium, and lithium hydroxides. Most are in the first and second groups of the periodic table. A superbase is extremely strong compared to sodium hydroxide and cannot be kept in an aqueous solution. Superbases are organized into organic, organometallic, and inorganic classes. Bases are used as insoluble catalysts in heterogeneous reactions and as catalysts in hydrogenation.

Some properties of salts are that they are formed from acid base reactions, are ionic compounds consisting of metallic and nonmetallic ions, dissociate in water, and are comprised of tightly bonded ions. Some common salts are sodium chloride ($NaCl$), sodium bisulfate, potassium dichromate ($K_2Cr_2O_7$), and calcium chloride ($CaCl_2$). Calcium chloride is used as a drying agent, and may be used to absorb moisture when freezing mixtures. Potassium nitrate (KNO_3) is used to make fertilizer and in the manufacture of explosives. Sodium nitrate ($NaNO_3$) is also used in the making of fertilizer. Baking soda (sodium bicarbonate) is a salt, as are Epsom salts [magnesium sulfate ($MgSO_4$)]. Salt and water can react to form a base and an acid. This is called a hydrolysis reaction.

A buffer is a solution whose pH remains relatively constant when a small amount of an acid or a base is added. It is usually made of a weak acid and its conjugate base (proton receiver) or one of its soluble salts. It can also be made of a weak base and its conjugate acid (proton donator) or one of its salts.

A constant pH is necessary in living cells because some living things can only live within a certain pH range. If that pH changes, the cells could die. Blood is an example of a buffer. A pKa is a measure of acid dissociation or the acid dissociation constant. Buffer solutions can help keep enzymes at the correct pH. They are also used in the fermentation process, in dyeing fabrics, and in the calibration of pH meters. An example of a buffer is HC_2H_3O (a weak acid) and $NaC_2H_3O_2$ (a salt containing the $C_2H_3O_2^-$ ion).

General Concepts

Lewis formulas: These show the bonding or nonbonding tendency of specific pairs of valence electrons. Lewis dot diagrams use dots to represent valence electrons. Dots are paired around an atom. When an atom forms a covalent bond with another atom, the elements share the dots as they would electrons. Double and triple bonds are indicated with additional adjacent dots. Methane (CH_4), for instance, would be shown as a C with 2 dots above, below, and to the right and left and an H next to each set of dots. In structural formulas, the dots are single lines.

Kekulé diagrams: Like Lewis dot diagrams, these are two-dimensional representations of chemical compounds. Covalent bonds are shown as lines between elements. Double and triple bonds are shown as two or three lines and unbonded valence electrons are shown as dots.

Molar mass: This refers to the mass of one mole of a substance (element or compound), usually measured in grams per mole (g/mol). This differs from molecular mass in that molecular mass is the mass of one molecule of a substance relative to the atomic mass unit (amu).

> **Review Video:** **Calculating the Molar Mass of a Substance**
> Visit mometrix.com/academy and enter code: 873284

Atomic mass unit (amu) is the smallest unit of mass, and is equal to 1/12 of the mass of the carbon isotope carbon-12. A mole (mol) is a measurement of molecular weight that is equal to the molecule's amu in grams. For example, carbon has an amu of 12, so a mole of carbon weighs 12 grams. One mole is equal to about 6.0221415×10^{23} elementary entities, which are usually atoms or molecules. This amount is also known as the Avogadro constant or Avogadro's number (N_A). Another way to say this is that one mole of a substance is the same as one Avogadro's number of that substance. One mole of chlorine, for example, is 6.0221415×10^{23} chlorine atoms. The charge on one mole of electrons is referred to as a Faraday.

The kinetic theory of gases assumes that gas molecules are small compared to the distances between them and that they are in constant random motion. The attractive and repulsive forces between gas molecules are negligible. Their kinetic energy does not change with time as long as the temperature remains the same. The higher the temperature is, the greater the motion will be. As the temperature of a gas increases, so does the kinetic energy of the molecules. In other words, gas will occupy a greater volume as the temperature is increased and a lesser volume as the temperature is decreased. In addition, the same amount of gas will occupy a greater volume as the temperature increases, but pressure remains constant. At any given temperature, gas molecules have the same average kinetic energy. The ideal gas law is derived from the kinetic theory of gases.

> **Review Video:** **Kinetic Molecular Theory**
> Visit mometrix.com/academy and enter code: 840030

Charles's law: This states that gases expand when they are heated. It is also known as the law of volumes.

Boyle's law: This states that gases contract when pressure is applied to them. It also states that if temperature remains constant, the relationship between absolute pressure and volume is inversely proportional. When one increases, the other decreases. Considered a specialized case of the ideal gas law, Boyle's law is sometimes known as the Boyle-Mariotte law.

The ideal gas law is used to explain the properties of a gas under ideal pressure, volume, and temperature conditions. It is best suited for describing monatomic gases (gases in which atoms are not bound together) and gases at high temperatures and low pressures. It is not well-suited for instances in which a gas or its components are close to their condensation point. All collisions are perfectly elastic and there are no intermolecular attractive forces at work. The ideal gas law is a way to explain and measure the macroscopic properties of matter. It can be derived from the kinetic theory of gases, which deals with the microscopic properties of matter. The equation for the ideal gas law is $PV = nRT$, where "P" is absolute pressure, "V" is absolute volume, and "T" is absolute temperature. "R" refers to the universal gas constant, which is 8.3145 J/mol Kelvin, and "n" is the number of moles.

Physics

Thermodynamics

Thermodynamics is a branch of physics that studies the conversion of energy into work and heat. It is especially concerned with variables such as temperature, volume, and pressure. Thermodynamic equilibrium refers to objects that have the same temperature because heat is transferred between them to reach equilibrium. Thermodynamics takes places within three different types of systems; open, isolated, and closed systems. Open systems are capable of interacting with a surrounding environment and can exchange heat, work (energy), and matter outside their system boundaries. A closed system can exchange heat and work, but not matter. An isolated system cannot exchange heat, work, or matter with its surroundings. Its total energy and mass stay the same. In physics, surrounding environment refers to everything outside a thermodynamic system (system). The terms "surroundings" and "environment" are also used. The term "boundary" refers to the division between the system and its surroundings.

The laws of thermodynamics are generalized principles dealing with energy and heat.

- The zeroth law of thermodynamics states that two objects in thermodynamic equilibrium with a third object are also in equilibrium with each other. Being in thermodynamic equilibrium basically means that different objects are at the same temperature.
- The first law deals with conservation of energy. It states that neither mass nor energy can be destroyed; only converted from one form to another.

> **Review Video: First Law of Thermodynamics**
> Visit mometrix.com/academy and enter code: 340643

- The second law states that the entropy (the amount of energy in a system that is no longer available for work or the amount of disorder in a system) of an isolated system can only increase. The second law also states that heat is not transferred from a lower-temperature system to a higher-temperature one unless additional work is done.

> **Review Video: The Second Law of Thermodynamics**
> Visit mometrix.com/academy and enter code: 251848

- The third law of thermodynamics states that as temperature approaches absolute zero, entropy approaches a constant minimum. It also states that a system cannot be cooled to absolute zero.

> **Review Video: Laws of Thermodynamics**
> Visit mometrix.com/academy and enter code: 253607

Thermal contact refers to energy transferred to a body by a means other than work. A system in thermal contact with another can exchange energy with it through the process of heat transfer. Thermal contact does not necessarily involve direct physical contact. Heat is energy that can be transferred from one body or system to another without work being done. Everything tends to become less organized and less useful over time (entropy). In all energy transfers, therefore, the overall result is that the heat is spread out so that objects are in thermodynamic equilibrium and the heat can no longer be transferred without additional work.

The laws of thermodynamics state that energy can be exchanged between physical systems as heat or work, and that systems are affected by their surroundings. It can be said that the total amount of energy in the universe is constant. The first law is mainly concerned with the conservation of energy and related concepts, which include the statement that energy can only be transferred or converted, not created or destroyed. The formula used to represent the first law is $\Delta U = Q - W$, where ΔU is the change in total internal energy of a system, Q is the heat added to the system, and W is the work done by the system. Energy can be transferred by conduction, convection, radiation, mass transfer, and other processes such as collisions in chemical and nuclear reactions. As transfers occur, the matter involved becomes less ordered and less useful. This tendency towards disorder is also referred to as entropy.

The second law of thermodynamics explains how energy can be used. In particular, it states that heat will not transfer spontaneously from a cold object to a hot object. Another way to say this is that heat transfers occur from higher temperatures to lower temperatures. Also covered under this law is the concept that systems not under the influence of external forces tend to become more disordered over time. This type of disorder can be expressed in terms of entropy.

Another principle covered under this law is that it is impossible to make a heat engine that can extract heat and convert it all to useful work. A thermal bottleneck occurs in machines that convert energy to heat and then use it to do work. These types of machines are less efficient than ones that are solely mechanical.

Conduction is a form of heat transfer that occurs at the molecular level. It is the result of molecular agitation that occurs within an object, body, or material while the material stays motionless. An example of this is when a frying pan is placed on a hot burner. At first, the handle is not hot. As the pan becomes hotter due to conduction, the handle eventually gets hot too. In this example, energy is being transferred down the handle toward the colder end because the higher speed particles collide with and transfer energy to the slower ones. When this happens, the original material becomes cooler and the second material becomes hotter until equilibrium is reached. Thermal conduction can also occur between two substances such as a cup of hot coffee and the colder surface it is placed on. Heat is transferred, but matter is not.

Convection refers to heat transfer that occurs through the movement or circulation of fluids (liquids or gases). Some of the fluid becomes or is hotter than the surrounding fluid, and is less dense. Heat is transferred away from the source of the heat to a cooler, denser area. Examples of convection are boiling water and the movement of warm and cold air currents in the atmosphere and the ocean. Forced convection occurs in convection ovens, where a fan helps circulate hot air.

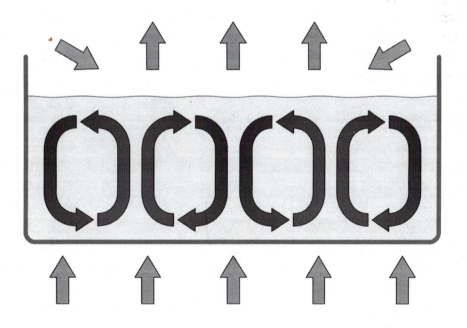

Radiation is heat transfer that occurs through the emission of electromagnetic waves, which carry energy away from the emitting object. All objects with temperatures above absolute zero radiate heat.

Temperature is a measurement of an object's stored heat energy. More specifically, temperature is the average kinetic energy of an object's particles. When the temperature of an object increases and its atoms move faster, kinetic energy also increases. Temperature is not energy since it changes and is not conserved. Thermometers are used to measure temperature.

There are three main scales for measuring temperature. Celsius uses the base reference points of water freezing at 0 degrees and boiling at 100 degrees. Fahrenheit uses the base reference points of water freezing at 32 degrees and boiling at 212 degrees. Celsius and Fahrenheit are both relative temperature scales since they use water as their reference point. The Kelvin temperature scale is an absolute temperature scale. Its zero mark corresponds to absolute zero. Water's freezing and boiling points are 273.15 Kelvin and 373.15 Kelvin, respectively. Where Celsius and Fahrenheit are measured is degrees, Kelvin does not use degree terminology.

- Converting Celsius to Fahrenheit: $°F = \frac{9}{5}°C + 32$
- Converting Fahrenheit to Celsius: $°C = \frac{5}{9}(°F - 32)$
- Converting Celsius to Kelvin: $K = °C + 273.15$
- Converting Kelvin to Celsius: $°C = K - 273.15$

Heat capacity, also known as thermal mass, refers to the amount of heat energy required to raise the temperature of an object, and is measured in Joules per Kelvin or Joules per degree Celsius. The equation for relating heat energy to heat capacity is $Q = C\Delta T$, where Q is the heat energy transferred, C is the heat capacity of the body, and ΔT is the change in the object's temperature. Specific heat capacity, also known as specific heat, is the heat capacity per unit mass. Every element and compound has its own specific heat. For example, it takes different amounts of heat energy to raise the temperature of the same amounts of magnesium and lead by one degree. The equation for relating heat energy to specific heat capacity is $Q = mc\Delta T$, where m represents the mass of the object, and c represents its specific heat capacity.

Some discussions of energy consider only two types of energy: kinetic energy (the energy of motion) and potential energy (which depends on relative position or orientation). There are, however, other types of energy. Electromagnetic waves, for example, are a type of energy contained by a field. Another type of potential energy is electrical energy, which is the energy it takes to pull apart positive and negative electrical charges. Chemical energy refers to the manner in which atoms form into molecules, and this energy can be released or absorbed when molecules regroup. Solar energy comes in the form of visible light and non-visible light, such as infrared and ultraviolet rays. Sound energy refers to the energy in sound waves.

Energy is constantly changing forms and being transferred back and forth. An example of a heat to mechanical energy transformation is a steam engine, such as the type used on a steam locomotive. A heat source such as coal is used to boil water. The steam produced turns a shaft, which eventually turns the wheels. A pendulum swinging is an example of both a kinetic to potential and a potential to kinetic energy transformation. When a pendulum is moved from its center point (the point at which it is closest to the ground) to the highest point before it returns, it is an example of a kinetic to potential transformation. When it swings from its highest point toward the center, it is considered a potential to kinetic transformation. The sum of the potential and kinetic energy is known as the total mechanical energy. Stretching a rubber band gives it potential energy. That potential energy becomes kinetic energy when the rubber band is released.

Motion and Force

Mechanics is the study of matter and motion, and the topics related to matter and motion, such as force, energy, and work. Discussions of mechanics will often include the concepts of vectors and scalars. Vectors are quantities with both magnitude and direction, while scalars have only magnitude. Scalar quantities include length, area, volume, mass, density, energy, work, and power. Vector quantities include displacement, direction, velocity, acceleration, momentum, and force.

Motion is a change in the location of an object, and is the result of an unbalanced net force acting on the object. Understanding motion requires the understanding of three basic quantities: displacement, velocity, and acceleration.

Displacement

When something moves from one place to another, it has undergone *displacement*. Displacement along a straight line is a very simple example of a vector quantity. If an object travels from position x = -5 cm to x = 5 cm, it has undergone a displacement of 10 cm. If it traverses the same path in the opposite direction, its displacement is -10 cm. A vector that spans the object's displacement in the direction of travel is known as a displacement vector.

> **Review Video: Displacement**
> Visit mometrix.com/academy and enter code: 236197

Velocity

There are two types of velocity to consider: *average velocity* and *instantaneous velocity*. Unless an object has a constant velocity or we are explicitly given an equation for the velocity, finding the instantaneous velocity of an object requires the use of calculus. If we want to calculate the *average velocity* of an object, we need to know two things: the displacement, or the distance it has covered, and the time it took to cover this distance. The formula for average velocity is simply the distance traveled divided by the time required. In other words, the average velocity is equal to the change in position divided by the change in time. Average velocity is a vector and will always point in the same direction as the displacement vector (since time is a scalar and always positive).

Acceleration

Acceleration is the change in the velocity of an object. On most test questions, the acceleration will be a constant value. Like position and velocity, acceleration is a vector quantity and will therefore have both magnitude and direction.

> **Review Video: Velocity and Acceleration**
> Visit mometrix.com/academy and enter code: 671849

Most motion can be explained by Newton's three laws of motion:

Newton's first law

An object at rest or in motion will remain at rest or in motion unless acted upon by an external force. This phenomenon is commonly referred to as inertia, the tendency of a body to remain in its present state of motion. In order for the body's state of motion to change, it must be acted on by an unbalanced force.

> **Review Video: Newton's First Law of Motion**
> Visit mometrix.com/academy and enter code: 590367

Newton's second law

An object's acceleration is directly proportional to the net force acting on the object, and inversely proportional to the object's mass. It is generally written in equation form $F = ma$, where F is the net force acting on a body, m is the mass of the body, and a is its acceleration. Note that since the mass is always a positive quantity, the acceleration is always in the same direction as the force.

> **Review Video: Newton's Second Law of Motion**
> Visit mometrix.com/academy and enter code: 737975

Newton's third law

For every force, there is an equal and opposite force. When a hammer strikes a nail, the nail hits the hammer just as hard. If we consider two objects, A and B, then we may express any contact between these two bodies with the equation $F_{AB} = -F_{BA}$, where the order of the subscripts denotes which body is exerting the force.

At first glance, this law might seem to forbid any movement at all since every force is being countered with an equal opposite force, but these equal opposite forces are acting on different bodies with different masses, so they will not cancel each other out.

> **Review Video: Newton's Third Law of Motion**
> Visit mometrix.com/academy and enter code: 838401

Energy

The two types of energy most important in mechanics are potential and kinetic energy. Potential energy is the amount of energy an object has stored within itself because of its position or orientation. There are many types of potential energy, but the most common is gravitational potential energy. It is the energy that an object has because of its height (h) above the ground. It can be calculated as $PE = mgh$, where m is the object's mass and g is the acceleration of gravity. Kinetic energy is the energy of an object in motion, and is calculated as $KE = mv^2/2$, where v is the magnitude of its velocity. When an object is dropped, its potential energy is converted into kinetic energy as it falls. These two equations can be used to calculate the velocity of an object at any point in its fall

> **Review Video: Potential and Kinetic Energy**
> Visit mometrix.com/academy and enter code: 491502

Work

Work can be thought of as the amount of energy expended in accomplishing some goal. The simplest equation for mechanical work (W) is $W = Fd$, where F is the force exerted and d is the displacement of the object on which the force is exerted. This equation requires that the force be applied in the same direction as the displacement. If this is not the case, then the work may be calculated as $W = Fd\cos(\theta)$, where θ is the angle between the force and displacement vectors. If force and displacement have the same direction, then work is positive; if they are in opposite directions, then work is negative; and if they are perpendicular, the work done by the force is zero.

As an example, if a man pushes a block horizontally across a surface with a constant force of 10 N for a distance of 20 m, the work done by the man is 200 N-m or 200 J. If instead the block is sliding and the man tries to slow its progress by pushing against it, his work done is -200 J, since he is pushing in the direction opposite the motion. If the man pushes vertically downward on the block while it slides, his work done is zero, since his force vector is perpendicular to the displacement vector of the block.

> **Review Video: Work**
> Visit mometrix.com/academy and enter code: 681834

Friction

Friction is a force that arises as a resistance to motion where two surfaces are in contact. The maximum magnitude of the frictional force (f) can be calculated as $f = F_c\mu$, where F_c is the contact force between the two objects and μ is a coefficient of friction based on the surfaces' material composition. Two types of friction are static and kinetic. To illustrate these concepts, imagine a book resting on a table. The force of its weight (W) is equal and opposite to the force of the table on the book, or the normal force (N). If we exert a small force (F) on the book, attempting to push it to one side, a frictional force (f) would arise, equal and opposite to our force. At this point, it is a *static frictional force* because the book is not moving. If we increase our force on the book, we will eventually cause it to move. At this point, the frictional force opposing us will be a *kinetic frictional force*. Generally, the kinetic frictional force is lower than static frictional force (because the frictional coefficient for static friction is larger), which means that the amount of force needed to maintain the movement of the book will be less than what was needed to start it moving.

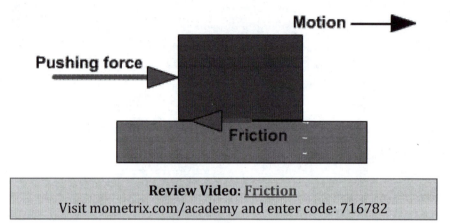

Gravitational force

Gravitational force is a universal force that causes every object to exert a force on every other object. The gravitational force between two objects can be described by the formula, $F = Gm_1m_2/r^2$, where m_1 and m_2 are the masses of two objects, r is the distance between them, and G is the gravitational constant, $G = 6.672 \times 10^{-11}$ N-m^2/kg^2.

In order for this force to have a noticeable effect, one or both of the objects must be extremely large, so the equation is generally only used in problems involving planetary bodies. For problems involving objects on the earth being affected by earth's gravitational pull, the force of gravity is simply calculated as $F = mg$, where g is 9.81 m/s^2 toward the ground.

Electrical force

Electrical force is a universal force that exists between any two electrically charged objects. Opposite charges attract one another and like charges repel one another. The magnitude of the force is directly proportional to the magnitude of the charges (q)and inversely proportional to the square of the distance (r) between the two objects: $F = kq_1q_2/r^2$, where $k = 9 \times 10^9$ N-m^2/C^2. Magnetic forces operate on a similar principle.

Buoyancy

Archimedes's principle states that a buoyant (upward) force on a submerged object is equal to the weight of the liquid displaced by the object. Water has a density of one gram per cubic centimeter. Anything that floats in water has a lower density, and anything that sinks has a higher density. This principle of buoyancy can also be used to calculate the volume of an irregularly shaped object. The mass of the object (m) minus its apparent mass in the water (m_a) divided by the density of water (ρ_w), gives the object's volume: $V = (m-m_a)/\rho_w$.

Machines

Simple machines include the inclined plane, lever, wheel and axle, and pulley. These simple machines have no internal source of energy. More complex or compound machines can be formed from them. Simple machines provide a force known as a mechanical advantage and make it easier to accomplish a task. The inclined plane enables a force less than the object's weight to be used to push an object to a greater height. A lever enables a multiplication of force. The wheel and axle allows for movement with less resistance. Single or double pulleys allows for easier direction of force. The wedge and screw are forms of the inclined plane. A wedge turns a smaller force working over a greater distance into a larger force. The screw is similar to an incline that is wrapped around a shaft.

A certain amount of work is required to move an object. The amount cannot be reduced, but by changing the way the work is performed a mechanical advantage can be gained. A certain amount of work is required to raise an object to a given vertical height. By getting to a given height at an angle, the effort required is reduced, but the distance that must be traveled to reach a given height is increased. An example of this is walking up a hill. One may take a direct, shorter, but steeper route, or one may take a more meandering, longer route that requires less effort. Examples of wedges include doorstops, axes, plows, zippers, and can openers.

A lever consists of a bar or plank and a pivot point or fulcrum. Work is performed by the bar, which swings at the pivot point to redirect the force. There are three types of levers: first, second, and third class. Examples of a first-class lever include balances, see-saws, nail extractors, and scissors (which also use wedges). In a second-class lever the fulcrum is placed at one end of the bar and the work is performed at the other end. The weight or load to be moved is in between. The closer to the fulcrum the weight is, the easier it is to move. Force is increased, but the distance it is moved is decreased. Examples include pry bars, bottle openers, nutcrackers, and wheelbarrows. In a third-class lever the fulcrum is at one end and the positions of the weight and the location where the work is performed are reversed. Examples include fishing rods, hammers, and tweezers.

> **Review Video: Levers**
> Visit mometrix.com/academy and enter code: 103910

The center of a wheel and axle can be likened to a fulcrum on a rotating lever. As it turns, the wheel moves a greater distance than the axle, but with less force. Obvious examples of the wheel and axle are the wheels of a car, but this type of simple machine can also be used to exert a greater force. For instance, a person can turn the handles of a winch to exert a greater force at the turning axle to move an object. Other examples include steering wheels, wrenches, faucets, waterwheels, windmills, gears, and belts. Gears work together to change a force. The four basic types of gears are spur, rack and pinion, bevel, and worm gears. The larger gear turns slower than the smaller, but exerts a greater force. Gears at angles can be used to change the direction of forces.

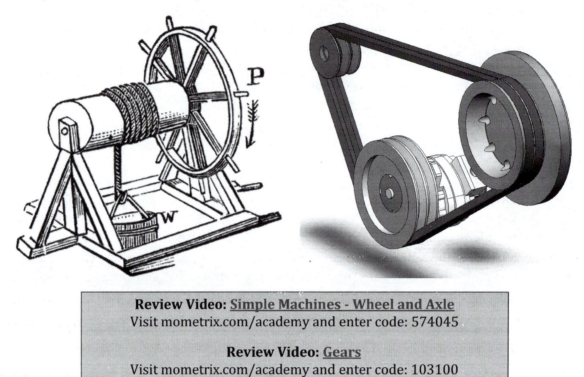

Review Video: Simple Machines - Wheel and Axle
Visit mometrix.com/academy and enter code: 574045

Review Video: Gears
Visit mometrix.com/academy and enter code: 103100

A single pulley consists of a rope or line that is run around a wheel. This allows force to be directed in a downward motion to lift an object. This does not decrease the force required, just changes its direction. The load is moved the same distance as the rope pulling it. When a combination pulley is used, such as a double pulley, the weight is moved half the distance of the rope pulling it. In this way, the work effort is doubled. Pulleys are never 100% efficient because of friction. Examples of pulleys include cranes, chain hoists, block and tackles, and elevators.

Review Video: Pulleys
Visit mometrix.com/academy and enter code: 103556

Electrical Charges

A glass rod and a plastic rod can illustrate the concept of static electricity due to friction. Both start with no charge. A glass rod rubbed with silk produces a positive charge, while a plastic rod rubbed with fur produces a negative charge. The electron affinity of a material is a property that helps determine how easily it can be charged by friction. Materials can be sorted by their affinity for electrons into a triboelectric series. Materials with greater affinities include celluloid, sulfur, and rubber. Materials with lower affinities include glass, rabbit fur, and asbestos. In the example of a glass rod and a plastic one, the glass rod rubbed with silk acquires a positive charge because glass has a lower affinity for electrons than silk. The electrons flow to the silk, leaving the rod with fewer electrons and a positive charge. When a plastic rod is rubbed with fur, electrons flow to the rod and result in a negative charge.

The attractive force between the electrons and the nucleus is called the electric force. A positive (+) charge or a negative (-) charge creates a field of sorts in the empty space around it, which is known as an electric field. The direction of a positive charge is away from it and the direction of a negative charge is towards it. An electron within the force of the field is pulled towards a positive charge because an electron has a negative charge. A particle with a positive charge is pushed away, or repelled, by another positive charge. Like charges repel each other and opposite charges attract. Lines of force show the paths of charges. Electric force between two objects is directly proportional to the product of the charge magnitudes and inversely proportional to the square of the distance between the two objects. Electric charge is measured with the unit Coulomb (C). It is the amount of charge moved in one second by a steady current of one ampere ($1C = 1A \times 1s$).

Insulators are materials that prevent the movement of electrical charges, while conductors are materials that allow the movement of electrical charges. This is because conductive materials have free electrons that can move through the entire volume of the conductor. This allows an external charge to change the charge distribution in the material. In induction, a neutral conductive material, such as a sphere, can become charged by a positively or negatively charged object, such as a rod. The charged object is placed close to the material without touching it. This produces a force on the free electrons, which will either be attracted to or repelled by the rod, polarizing (or separating) the charge. The sphere's electrons will flow into or out of it when touched by a ground. The sphere is now charged. The charge will be opposite that of the charging rod.

Charging by conduction is similar to charging by induction, except that the material transferring the charge actually touches the material receiving the charge. A negatively or positively charged object is touched to an object with a neutral charge. Electrons will either flow into or out of the neutral object and it will become charged. Insulators cannot be used to conduct charges. Charging by conduction can also be called charging by contact.

> **Review Video: Charging by Conduction**
> Visit mometrix.com/academy and enter code: 502661

The law of conservation of charge states that the total number of units before and after a charging process remains the same. No electrons have been created. They have just been moved around. The removal of a charge on an object by conduction is called grounding.

Circuits

Electric potential, or electrostatic potential or voltage, is an expression of potential energy per unit of charge. It is measured in volts (V) as a scalar quantity. The formula used is $V = E/Q$, where V is voltage, E is electrical potential energy, and Q is the charge. Voltage is typically discussed in the context of electric potential difference between two points in a circuit. Voltage can also be thought of as a measure of the rate at which energy is drawn from a source in order to produce a flow of electric charge.

Electric current is the sustained flow of electrons that are part of an electric charge moving along a path in a circuit. This differs from a static electric charge, which is a constant non-moving charge rather than a continuous flow. The rate of flow of electric charge is expressed using the ampere (amp or A) and can be measured using an ammeter. A current of 1 ampere means that 1 coulomb of charge passes through a given area every second. Electric charges typically only move from areas of high electric potential to areas of low electric potential. To get charges to flow into a high potential area, you must to connect it to an area of higher potential, by introducing a battery or other voltage source.

Electric currents experience resistance as they travel through a circuit. Different objects have different levels of resistance. The ohm (Ω) is the measurement unit of electric resistance. The symbol is the Greek letter omega. Ohm's Law, which is expressed as $I = V/R$, states that current flow (I, measured in amps) through an object is equal to the potential difference from one side to the other (V, measured in volts) divided by resistance (R, measured in ohms). An object with a higher resistance will have a lower current flow through it given the same potential difference.

Movement of electric charge along a path between areas of high electric potential and low electric potential, with a resistor or load device between them, is the definition of a simple circuit. It is a closed conducting path between the high and low potential points, such as the positive and negative terminals on a battery. One example of a circuit is the flow from one terminal of a car battery to the other. The electrolyte solution of water and sulfuric acid provides work in chemical form to start the flow. A frequently used classroom example of circuits involves using a D cell (1.5 V) battery, a small light bulb, and a piece of copper wire to create a circuit to light the bulb.

> **Review Video: Electrical Circuits**
> Visit mometrix.com/academy and enter code: 472696

Magnets

A magnet is a piece of metal, such as iron, steel, or magnetite (lodestone) that can affect another substance within its field of force that has like characteristics. Magnets can either attract or repel other substances. Magnets have two poles: north and south. Like poles repel and opposite poles (pairs of north and south) attract. The magnetic field is a set of invisible lines representing the paths of attraction and repulsion. Magnetism can occur naturally, or ferromagnetic materials can be magnetized. Certain matter that is magnetized can retain its magnetic properties indefinitely and become a permanent magnet. Other matter can lose its magnetic properties. For example, an iron nail can be temporarily magnetized by stroking it repeatedly in the same direction using one pole of another magnet. Once magnetized, it can attract or repel other magnetically inclined materials, such as paper clips. Dropping the nail repeatedly will cause it to lose its charge.

The motions of subatomic structures (nuclei and electrons) produce a magnetic field. It is the direction of the spin and orbit that indicate the direction of the field. The strength of a magnetic field is known as the magnetic moment. As electrons spin and orbit a nucleus, they produce a magnetic field. Pairs of electrons that spin and orbit in opposite directions cancel each other out, creating a net magnetic field of zero. Materials that have an unpaired electron are magnetic. Those with a weak attractive force are referred to as paramagnetic materials, while ferromagnetic materials have a strong attractive force. A diamagnetic material has electrons that are paired, and therefore does not typically have a magnetic moment. There are, however, some diamagnetic materials that have a weak magnetic field.

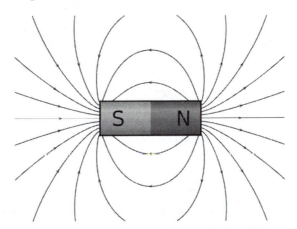

A magnetic field can be formed not only by a magnetic material, but also by electric current flowing through a wire. When a coiled wire is attached to the two ends of a battery, for example, an electromagnet can be formed by inserting a ferromagnetic material such as an iron bar within the coil. When electric current flows through the wire, the bar becomes a magnet. If there is no current, the magnetism is lost. A magnetic domain occurs when the magnetic fields of atoms are grouped and aligned. These groups form what can be thought of as miniature magnets within a material. This is what happens when an object like an iron nail is temporarily magnetized. Prior to magnetization, the organization of atoms and their various polarities are somewhat random with respect to where the north and south poles are pointing. After magnetization, a significant percentage of the poles are lined up in one direction, which is what causes the magnetic force exerted by the material.

> **Review Video: Magnets**
> Visit mometrix.com/academy and enter code: 570803

Waves

Waves have energy and can transfer energy when they interact with matter. Although waves transfer energy, they do not transport matter. They are a disturbance of matter that transfers energy from one particle to an adjacent particle. There are many types of waves, including sound, seismic, water, light, micro, and radio waves. The two basic categories of waves are mechanical and electromagnetic. Mechanical waves are those that transmit energy through matter. Electromagnetic waves can transmit energy through a vacuum. A transverse wave provides a good illustration of the features of a wave, which include crests, troughs, amplitude, and wavelength. There are a number of important attributes of waves.

Frequency is a measure of how often particles in a medium vibrate when a wave passes through the medium with respect to a certain point or node. Usually measured in Hertz (Hz), frequency might refer to cycles per second, vibrations per second, or waves per second. One Hz is equal to one cycle per second.

Period is a measure of how long it takes to complete a cycle. It is the inverse of frequency; where frequency is measure in cycles per second, period can be thought of as seconds per cycle, though it is measured in units of time only.

Speed refers to how fast or slow a wave travels. It is measured in terms of distance divided by time. While frequency is measured in terms of cycles per second, speed might be measured in terms of meters per second.

Amplitude is the maximum amount of displacement of a particle in a medium from its rest position, and corresponds to the amount of energy carried by the wave. High energy waves have greater amplitudes; low energy waves have lesser amplitudes. Amplitude is a measure of a wave's strength.

Rest position, also called equilibrium, is the point at which there is neither positive nor negative displacement. Crest, also called the peak, is the point at which a wave's positive or upward displacement from the rest position is at its maximum. Trough, also called a valley, is the point at which a wave's negative or downward displacement from the rest position is at its maximum. A wavelength is one complete wave cycle. It could be measured from crest to crest, trough to trough, rest position to rest position, or any point of a wave to the corresponding point on the next wave.

Sound is a pressure disturbance that moves through a medium in the form of mechanical waves, which transfer energy from one particle to the next. Sound requires a medium to travel through, such as air, water, or other matter since it is the vibrations that transfer energy to adjacent particles, not the actual movement of particles over a great distance. Sound is transferred through the movement of atomic particles, which can be atoms or molecules. Waves of sound energy move outward in all directions from the source. Sound waves consist of compressions (particles are forced together) and rarefactions (particles move farther apart and their density decreases). A wavelength consists of one compression and one rarefaction. Different sounds have different wavelengths. Sound is a form of kinetic energy.

The electromagnetic spectrum is defined by frequency (f) and wavelength (λ). Frequency is typically measured in hertz and wavelength is usually measured in meters. Because light travels at a fairly constant speed, frequency is inversely proportional to wavelength, a relationship expressed by the formula $f = c/\lambda$, where c is the speed of light (about 300 million meters per second). Frequency multiplied by wavelength equals the speed of the wave; for electromagnetic waves, this is the speed of light, with some variance for the medium in which it is traveling. Electromagnetic waves include (from largest to smallest wavelength) radio waves, microwaves, infrared radiation (radiant heat), visible light, ultraviolet radiation, x-rays, and gamma rays. The energy of electromagnetic waves is carried in packets that have a magnitude inversely proportional to the wavelength. Radio waves have a range of wavelengths, from about 10^{-3} to 10^5 meters, while their frequencies range from 10^3 to about 10^{11} Hz.

> **Review Video:** <u>Electromagnetic Radiation Waves</u>
> Visit mometrix.com/academy and enter code: 135307

Atoms and molecules can gain or lose energy only in particular, discrete amounts. Therefore, they can absorb and emit light only at wavelengths that correspond to these amounts. Using a process known as spectroscopy, these characteristic wavelengths can be used to identify substances.

Light is the portion of the electromagnetic spectrum that is visible because of its ability to stimulate the retina. It is absorbed and emitted by electrons, atoms, and molecules that move from one energy level to another. Visible light interacts with matter through molecular electron excitation (which occurs in the human retina) and through plasma oscillations (which occur in metals). Visible light is between ultraviolet and infrared light on the spectrum. The wavelengths of visible light cover a range from 380 nm (violet) to 760 nm (red). Different wavelengths correspond to different colors. The human brain interprets or perceives visible light, which is emitted from the sun and other stars, as color. For example, when the entire wavelength reaches the retina, the brain perceives the color white. When no part of the wavelength reaches the retina, the brain perceives the color black.

When light waves encounter an object, they are either reflected, transmitted, or absorbed. If the light is reflected from the surface of the object, the angle at which it contacts the surface will be the same as the angle at which it leaves, on the other side of the perpendicular. If the ray of light is perpendicular to the surface, it will be reflected back in the direction from which it came. When light is transmitted through the object, its direction may be altered upon entering the object. This is known as refraction. The degree to which the light is refracted depends on the speed at which light travels in the object. Light that is neither reflected nor transmitted will be absorbed by the surface and stored as heat energy. Nearly all instances of light hitting an object will involve a combination of two or even all three of these.

When light waves are refracted, or bent, an image can appear distorted. Sound waves and water waves can also be refracted. Diffraction refers to the bending of waves around small objects and the spreading out of waves past small openings. The narrower the opening, the greater the level of diffraction will be. Larger wavelengths also increase diffraction. A diffraction grating can be created by placing a number of slits close together, and is used more frequently than a prism to separate light. Different wavelengths are diffracted at different angles. The particular color of an object depends upon what is absorbed and what is transmitted or reflected.

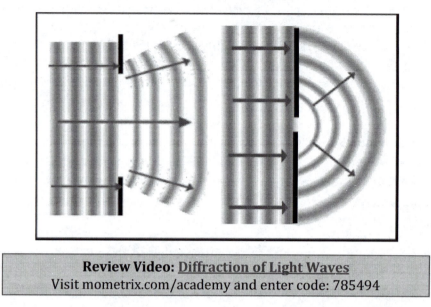

Review Video: <u>Diffraction of Light Waves</u>
Visit mometrix.com/academy and enter code: 785494

For example, a leaf consists of chlorophyll molecules, the atoms of which absorb all wavelengths of the visible light spectrum except for green, which is why a leaf appears green. Certain wavelengths of visible light can be absorbed when they interact with matter. Wavelengths that are not absorbed can be transmitted by transparent materials or reflected by opaque materials.

The various properties of light have numerous real life applications. For example, polarized sunglasses have lenses that help reduce glare, while non-polarized sunglasses reduce the total amount of light that reaches the eyes. Polarized lenses consist of a chemical film of molecules aligned in parallel. This allows the lenses to block wavelengths of light that are intense, horizontal, and reflected from smooth, flat surfaces. The "fiber" in fiber optics refers to a tube or pipe that channels light. Because of the composition of the fiber, light can be transmitted greater distances before losing the signal. The fiber consists of a core, cladding, and a coating. Fibers are bundled, allowing for the transmission of large amounts of data.

Part IV- Judgment and Comprehension in Practical Nursing Situations

The questions in this part will describe a work situation and ask you how you should respond. Don't worry; you won't be tested over things you haven't learned yet in nursing school. These questions will deal with topics like how to handle unruly patients or irritating coworkers, rather than testing your knowledge of diseases or interventions. These questions can all be answered by applying a good measure of common sense.

If the correct answer is not obvious after reading the question and the answer choices, begin eliminating answer choices using the following steps:

1. Patient safety: Eliminate any choices that might cause harm to the patient.
2. Personal safety: Eliminate any choices that might cause harm to you.
3. Patient emotions: Eliminate any choices that might offend the patient or the patient's friends/relatives, particularly if there is a cultural or ethnic component to the situation.
4. Coworker relations: Eliminate any choices that are unnecessarily confrontational or that would be likely to cause workplace hostility or animosity.

In most cases, this method should eliminate all but the correct answer.

Many of the questions will include a choice to involve your supervisor. While it may be tempting to select this choice frequently, you are expected to be able to handle your own problems most of the time. Generally, you should only select a choice that involves your supervisor if there is a problem that cannot be handled tactfully without him or her.

Part V. – Vocational Adjustment Index

This is a mini-test that evaluates your opinions and attitudes related to the nursing profession and practice as a professional. You cannot prepare for this section of the exam. You will be asked questions on quality of care, delivery of services, and patient rights. Moreover, the goal of this mini-test is to determine your opinions about professional care. If you answer with "extreme" points of view, you will not be scored well on this assessment.

PSB Practical Nursing Practice Test

Academic Aptitude

Verbal

In the following sets of words, choose the word that is most different in meaning from the others.

1. a. Expand   b. Contract   c. Shrink   d. Diminish   e. Lessen
2. a. Abhor   b. Adore   c. Despise   d. Hate   e. Deplore
3. a. Trite   b. Cliché   c. Original   d. Overused   e. Commonplace
4. a. Bicker   b. Argue   c. Quarrel   d. Cooperate   e. Disagree
5. a. Pandemonium   b. Chaos   c. Excitement   d. Disarray   e. Harmony
6. a. Somber   b. Gleeful   c. Serious   d. Sad   e. Gloomy
7. a. Apprehension b. Trepidation   c. Optimism   d. Dread   e. Anxiety
8. a. Dismal   b. Dreary   c. Bleak   d. Cheery   e. Depressing
9. a. Fortunate   b. Hapless   c. Unlucky   d. Tragic   e. Doomed
10. a. Disperse   b. Thin   c. Collect   d. Dissipate   e. Scatter
11. a. Oblivious   b. Clueless   c. Aware   d. Heedless   e. Ignorant
12. a. Distraught   b. Alarmed   c. Agitated   d. Tranquil   e. Distracted
13. a. Bedlam   b. Confusion   c. Havoc   d. Uproar   e. Order
14. a. Ambiguous   b. Clear   c. Vague   d. Arcane   e. Cryptic
15. a. Invite   b. Avert   c. Evade   d. Prevent   e. Elude
16. a. Unique   b. Mundane   c. Ordinary   d. Quotidian   e. Pedestrian
17. a. Perpetual   b. Constant   c. Occasional   d. Ceaseless   e. Running
18. a. Vexing   b. Gratifying   c. Irritating   d. Annoying   e. Aggravating
19. a. Sagacious   b. Wise   c. Knowing   d. Ignorant   e. Astute
20. a. Audacious   b. Bold   c. Brash   d. Rude   e. Humble
21. a. Deriding   b. Approving   c. Praising   d. Favoring   e. Commending
22. a. Stealthy   b. Secretive   c. Sneaky   d. Sly   e. Transparent
23. a. Impudent   b. Impertinent   c. Respectful   d. Rude   e. Sassy
24. a. Blissful   b. Blithe   c. Jubilant   d. Aggrieved   e. Jocund
25. a. Gaunt   b. Plump   c. Haggard   d. Wasted   e. Skinny
26. a. Unassuming   b. Haughty   c. Superior   d. Lofty   e. Presumptuous
27. a. Blasphemous b. Reverent   c. Profane   d. Impious   e. Sacrilegious
28. a. Heretic   b. Renegade   c. Believer   d. Defector   e. Dissident
29. a. Cynical   b. Trusting   c. Skeptical   d. Suspicious   e. Pessimistic
30. a. Agape   b. Anticipating c. Eager   d. Unmoved   e. Agog

- 93 -

Arithmetic

1. 236
   +301
       a. 505
       b. 507
       c. 535
       d. 537

2. 4,307
   +1,864
       a. 5,161
       b. 5,271
       c. 6,171
       d. 6,271

3. If $a = 3$ and $b = -2$, what is the value of $a^2 + 3ab - b^2$?
       a. 5
       b. -13
       c. -4
       d. -20

4. 356
   - 167
       a. 189
       b. 198
       c. 211
       d. 298

5. 5,306
   -3,487
       a. 1,181
       b. 1,819
       c. 2,119
       d. 2,189

6. 34 is what percent of 80?
       a. 34%
       b. 40%
       c. 42.5%
       d. 44.5%

7. 707

   x 17

    a. 12,019
    b. 12,049
    c. 17,019
    d. 17,049

8. $7\overline{)917}$

    a. 131
    b. 131 R4
    c. 145
    d. 145 R4

9. Factor the following expression: $x^2 + x - 12$

    a. $(x - 4)(x + 4)$
    b. $(x - 2)(x + 6)$
    c. $(x + 6)(x - 2)$
    d. $(x + 4)(x - 3)$

10. $\frac{38}{100}$ as a decimal

    a. 0.38
    b. 0.038
    c. 3.8
    d. 0.0038

11.   6.8

      11.3

  +   0.06

    a. 17.16
    b. 17.70
    c. 18.16
    d. 18.70

12. The average of six numbers is 4. If the average of two of those numbers is 2, what is the average of the other four numbers?

    a. 5
    b. 6
    c. 7
    d. 8

13. Which numeral is in the thousandths place in 0.3874?

    a. 3
    b. 8
    c. 7
    d. 4

14. 0.58 - 0.39=

    a. 0.19

    b. 1.9

    c. 0.29

    d. 2.9

15. Solve: 0.25 x 0.03 =

    a. 75

    b. 0.075

    c. 0.75

    d. 0.0075

16. $3\frac{1}{8} + 6 + \frac{3}{7} =$

    a. $9\frac{31}{56}$

    b. $9\frac{1}{2}$

    c. $9\frac{21}{56}$

    d. $9\frac{7}{8}$

17. $4\frac{1}{7} - 2\frac{1}{2} =$

    a. $2\frac{5}{14}$

    b. $1\frac{5}{14}$

    c. $1\frac{9}{14}$

    d. $2\frac{9}{14}$

18. $1\frac{1}{4} \times 3\frac{2}{5} \times 1\frac{2}{3} =$

    a. $7\frac{1}{12}$

    b. $5\frac{5}{6}$

    c. $6\frac{7}{12}$

    d. $8\frac{11}{15}$

19. How many 3-inch segments can a 4.5-yard line be divided into?

    a. 15

    b. 45

    c. 54

    d. 64

20. Reduce $\frac{14}{98}$ to lowest terms.

    a. $\frac{7}{49}$

    b. $\frac{2}{14}$

    c. $\frac{1}{7}$

    d. $\frac{3}{8}$

21. Thirty six hundredths as a percent.

    a. 36%

    b. 0.36%

    c. 0.036%

    d. 3.6%

22. 40% of 900

    a. 280

    b. 340

    c. 360

    d. 420

23. Sheila, Janice, and Karen, working together at the same rate, can complete a job in 3 1/3 days. Working at the same rate, how much of the job could Janice and Karen do in one day?

    a. $\frac{1}{5}$

    b. $\frac{1}{4}$

    c. $\frac{1}{3}$

    d. $\frac{1}{9}$

24. Three eighths of forty equals:

    a. 15

    b. 20

    c. 22

    d. 24

25. 6% of 25

    a. .3

    b. 1.5

    c. 3.0

    d. 15

26. Ratio of 4 to 16 = (?)%

    a. 2

    b. 4

    c. 12

    d. 25

27. $4^6 \div 2^8 =$

    a. 2

    b. 8

    c. 16

    d. 32

28. 30% as a reduced common fraction

    a. $\frac{30}{100}$

    b. $\frac{1}{30}$

    c. $\frac{23}{10}$

    d. $\frac{3}{10}$

29. 37% as a decimal

    a. .0037

    b. .037

    c. .37

    d. 3.7

30. $-4a + 6a + 2a$

    a. $4a$

    b. $-4a$

    c. $8a$

    d. $12a$

Nonverbal

For each question, there is a relationship between the first two figures presented, and then a third figure is presented. Find the answer choice that relates to the third figure in the same way that the first two figures are related.

1. ▣ is to ▭ as ◖I◗ is to? a. ○ b. ▭ c. ◉ d. ▣ e. ◫

2. ▯ is to ◻ as ◯ is to? a. △ b. ○ c. ⬭ d. ▱ e. ◺

3. ◉ is to ○ as ▣ is to? a. ○ b. ▭ c. ◻ d. ▣ e. ◫

4. ▯ is to ◿ as ○ is to? a. ◿ b. ▯ c. ⬭ d. ◖ e. △

5. ◎ is to ▭ as (is to? a. ▣ b. ∪ c. ⬭ d. ◿ e. ⌐

6. △ is to ▽ as ⌒ is to? a. ◁ b. ▷ c. ◖ d. ⌣ e. ○

7. ✦ is to ☆ as ✡ is to? a. △ b. ✖ c. ✹ d. ✴ e. ▽

8. ⅅ is to ○ as ▷ is to? a. ▽ b. ◇ c. ⅅ d. ▭ e. △

9. ▥ is to ▤ as ◍ is to? a. ⊖ b. ▭ c. ○ d. ◍ e. ▨

10. ◇ is to ◈ as ○ is to? a. ◈ b. ⬤ c. ◎ d. ◇ e. ○

11. ✻ is to ✸ as ☺ is to? a. ☆ b. ○ c. ☺ d. ○ e. ✪

12. ⤴ is to ⤶ as ⬆ is to? a. ⬇ b. ⬅ c. ➡ d. ⬍ e. ◿

13. ✚ is to ∅ as ▤ is to? a. ▭ b. ✚ c. ◎ d. ◿ e. ⌐

14. ◍ to ○ as ▦ is to? a. ▲ b. ▦ c. ▯ d. ▭ e. ○

- 99 -

15. is to as is to? a. b. c. d. e.

16. is to as is to? a. b. c. d. e.

17. is to as is to? a. b. c. d. e.

18. is to as is to? a. b. c. d. e.

19. is to as is to? a. b. c. d. e.

20. is to as is to? a. b. c. d. e.

16. is to as is to? a. b. c. d. e.

17. is to as is to? a. b. c. d. e.

18. is to as is to? a. b. c. d. e.

19. is to as is to? a. b. c. d. e.

20. is to as is to? a. b. c. d. e.

21. is to as is to? a. b. c. d. e.

- 100 -

22. ▭⟩ is to ⟩⟩ as ⟩⟩ is to? a. ⟨⟨ b. ⟨⟨ c. ⟩ d. ⬯ e. ⬠

23. ⌐↓ is to └↓ as ↑ is to? a. ↑ b. → c. ← d. ↘ e. ↓

24. ⌐↑ is to └↑ as ∫ is to? a. ↗ b. ↕ c. ↓ d. ↙ e. ⌐∫

25. ✛ is to ⇕ as ⇑ is to? a. ⇒ b. ⇓ c. ⇑ d. ⇔ e. ⬆

26. ◎ is to ◯ as ⊓ is to? a. ○ b. ◉ c. ⊓ d. ⊔ e. ⊡

27. ◇ is to ◈ as ◎ is to? a. ○ b. ◉ c. ◇ d. ⊙ e. ◯

28. ◯ is to ☾ as ▢ is to? a. ☽ b. ◖ c. ◪ d. ▯ e. ⌐

29. ⏢ is to ⬓ as ⬤ is to? a. ◖ b. ◯ c. ◁ d. ▷ e. ◗

30. ⬿ is to ⬡ as △ is to? a. ◇ b. ▽ c. ▯ d. ⬭ e. ▽

Spelling

Each question gives three different spellings of a word. Two are incorrect and one is correct. Select the choice from each set of three that is spelled correctly.

1. a. separate   b. seperate   c. sepparate
2. a. nucular   b. nuclear   c. nuculear
3. a. fermiliar   b. farmiliar   c. familiar
4. a. sacrilegious   b. sacreligious   c. sacraligious
5. a. aggitated   b. agittated   c. agitated
6. a. orientated   b. oriented   c. oreinted
7. a. indispensible   b. indespensible   c. indispensable
8. a. similar   b. simular   c. similiar
9. a. atitude   b. attitude   c. atittude
10. a. abreviate   b. abbreviate   c. abreeviate
11. a. absorb   b. apsorb   c. abzorb
12. a. acumulate   b. acummulate   c. accumulate
13. a. airial   b. aireal   c. aerial
14. a. comedian   b. commedian   c. comedien
15. a. ashphalt   b. asphalt   c. aspalt
16. a. forceable   b. forcible   c. forceble
17. a. anicdote   b. antecdote   c. anecdote
18. a. flexible   b. flexable   c. flexiable
19. a. defendant   b. defendent   c. difendent
20. a. plainteff   b. plaintif   c. plaintiff
21. a. idiocincrasy   b. idiosyncrasy   c. idiosincracy
22. a. hazardous   b. hazerdous   c. hazzardous
23. a. horific   b. horrific   c. horriffic
24. a. hansome   b. handsom   c. handsome
25. a. liaison   b. liason   c. leiaison
26. a. galexy   b. galaxy   c. gallaxy
27. a. attorneys   b. atorneys   c. attornys
28. a. asteriks   b. asterix   c. asterisk
29. a. equalibrium   b. equilibrum   c. equilibrium
30. a. brilliance   b. brillance   c. briliance
31. a. blanche   b. blanch   c. blance
32. a. ecstasy   b. extasy   c. ecstacy
33. a. deppreciate   b. depreciate   c. deappreciate
34. a. terpitude   b. turpittude   c. turpitude
35. a. oposite   b. opposite   c. opossite
36. a. tyrrany   b. tyrranny   c. tyranny
37. a. schism   b. scism   c. shism
38. a. scedule   b. shedule   c. schedule
39. a. incandescent   b. incandesent   c. incandecent
40. a. teriffic   b. terrific   c. terriffic
41. a. homogeneize   b. homogenize   c. homoginise
42. a. sieve   b. seive   c. sive
43. a. truely   b. truley   c. truly
44. a. sincerely   b. sincerly   c. sinceerly
45. a. transeint   b. transient   c. transhent

46. a. sedition   b. sidition   c. sadition
47. a. theives   b. thiefs   c. thieves
48. a. vengance   b. vengeance   c. vengence
49. a. nilon   b. nylon   c. nyllon
50. a. unnacceptable   b. unaceptible   c. unacceptable
51. a. deficit   b. defecit   c. defficit
52. a. disaproval   b. disapproval   c. dissaproval
53. a. diffidence   b. difidence   c. diffedince
54. a. picknicking   b. picnicing   c. picnicking
55. a. oreggano   b. oreganno   c. oregano
56. a. batchelor   b. bachelor   c. bachler
57. a. indelible   b. indelable   c. indellible
58. a. dyurnal   b. diurnal   c. dayernal
59. a. impatience   b. impatiense   c. empatiance
60. a. parlament   b. parliment   c. parliament

Natural Science

1. What is the name for any substance that stimulates the production of antibodies?

    a. collagen
    b. hemoglobin
    c. lymph
    d. antigen

2. Which of the following correctly lists the cellular hierarchy from the simplest to the most complex structure?

    a. tissue, cell, organ, organ system, organism
    b. organism, organ system, organ, tissue, cell
    c. organ system, organism, organ, tissue, cell
    d. cell, tissue, organ, organ system, organism

3. If a cell is placed in a hypertonic solution, what will happen to the cell?

    a. It will swell.
    b. It will shrink.
    c. It will stay the same.
    d. It does not affect the cell.

4. Which group of major parts and organs make up the immune system?

    a. lymphatic system, spleen, tonsils, thymus, and bone marrow
    b. brain, spinal cord, and nerve cells
    c. heart, veins, arteries, and capillaries
    d. nose, trachea, bronchial tubes, lungs, alveolus, and diaphragm

5. The rate of a chemical reaction depends on all of the following except

    a. temperature
    b. surface area.
    c. presence of catalysts.
    d. amount of mass lost.

6. Which of the answer choices provided best defines the following statement?

For a given mass and constant temperature, an inverse relationship exists between the volume and pressure of a gas.

    a. Ideal Gas Law
    b. Boyle's Law
    c. Charles' Law
    d. Stefan-Boltzmann Law

7. Which of the following statements correctly compares prokaryotic and eukaryotic cells?

    a. Prokaryotic cells have a true nucleus, eukaryotic cells do not.
    b. Both prokaryotic and eukaryotic cells have a membrane.
    c. Prokaryotic cells do not contain membrane-bound organelles, eukaryotic cells do.
    d. Prokaryotic cells are more complex than eukaryotic cells.

8. What is the role of ribosomes?

    a. make proteins

    b. waste removal

    c. transport

    d. storage

9. If an organism is *AaBb*, which of the following combinations in the gametes is impossible?

    a. AB

    b. aa

    c. aB

    d. Ab

10. What is the oxidation number of hydrogen in CaH_2?

    a. +1

    b. –1

    c. 0

    d. +2

11. Which hormone stimulates milk production in the breasts during lactation?

    a. norepinephrine

    b. antidiuretic hormone

    c. prolactin

    d. oxytocin

12. What is the typical result of mitosis in humans?

    a. two diploid cells

    b. two haploid cells

    c. four diploid cells

    d. four haploid cells

13. Which of the following does *not* exist as a diatomic molecule?

    a. boron

    b. fluorine

    c. oxygen

    d. nitrogen

14. Which of the following structures has the lowest blood pressure?

    a. arteries

    b. arteriole

    c. venule

    d. vein

15. How does water affect the temperature of a living thing?

    a. Water increases temperature.

    b. Water keeps temperature stable.

    c. Water decreases temperature.

    d. Water does not affect temperature.

16. What is another name for aqueous HI?

    a. hydroiodate acid
    b. hydrogen monoiodide
    c. hydrogen iodide
    d. hydriodic acid

17. Which of the heart chambers is the most muscular?

    a. left atrium
    b. right atrium
    c. left ventricle
    d. right ventricle

18. Which of the following is *not* a product of the Krebs cycle?

    a. carbon dioxide
    b. oxygen
    c. adenosine triphosphate (ATP)
    d. energy carriers

19. What is the name for the reactant that is entirely consumed by the reaction?

    a. limiting reactant
    b. reducing agent
    c. reaction intermediate
    d. reagent

20. Which part of the brain interprets sensory information?

    a. cerebrum
    b. hindbrain
    c. cerebellum
    d. medulla oblongata

21. What kind of bond connects sugar and phosphate in DNA?

    a. hydrogen
    b. ionic
    c. covalent
    d. overt

22. What is the mass (in grams) of 7.35 mol water?

    a. 10.7 g
    b. 18 g
    c. 132 g
    d. 180.6 g

23. Which of the following proteins is produced by cartilage?

    a. actin
    b. estrogen
    c. collagen
    d. myosin

24. How are lipids different than other organic molecules?

    a. They are indivisible.
    b. They are not water soluble.
    c. They contain zinc.
    d. They form long proteins.

25. Which of the following orbitals is the last to fill?

    a. 1s
    b. 3s
    c. 4p
    d. 6s

26. Which component of the nervous system is responsible for lowering the heart rate?

    a. central nervous system
    b. sympathetic nervous system
    c. parasympathetic nervous system
    d. distal nervous system

27. Which of the following is *not* a steroid?

    a. cholesterol
    b. estrogen
    c. testosterone
    d. hemoglobin

28. What is the name of the binary molecular compound NO_5?

    a. cnitro pentoxide
    b. ammonium pentoxide
    c. nitrogen pentoxide
    d. pentnitrogen oxide

29. In which of the following muscle types are the filaments arranged in a disorderly manner?

    a. cardiac
    b. smooth
    c. skeletal
    d. rough

30. Which hormone is produced by the pineal gland?

    a. insulin
    b. testosterone
    c. melatonin
    d. epinephrine

31. Make the following metric conversion: 5 decimeters = _____ decameters

    a. 0.5
    b. 0.05
    c. 50
    d. 500

32. Which of the data sets could be plotted on a pie chart?

    a. The total population of the top five largest U.S. cities.
    b. The incubation period of a penguin colony as it relates to hours of daylight.
    c. The distribution of weight among players of a football team.
    d. The percent of vegetation cover and precipitation rates in different national parks.

33. Which of the following processes uses electrical charges to separate substances?

    a. Spectrophotometry
    b. Chromatography
    c. Centrifugation
    d. Electrophoresis

34. When using a light microscope, how is the total magnification determined?

    a. By multiplying the ocular lens power times the objective being used.
    b. By looking at the objective you are using only.
    c. By looking at the ocular lens power only.
    d. By multiplying the objective you are using times two.

35. When undergoing a dissection in class, which of the following procedures is incorrect?

    a. Rinse the specimen before handling.
    b. Dispose of harmful chemicals according to district regulations.
    c. Decaying specimens are never permitted but unknown specimens are sometimes permitted.
    d. Students with open sores on their hands that cannot be covered should be excused from the dissection.

36. After a science laboratory exercise, some solutions remain unused and are left over. What should be done with these solutions?

    a. Dispose of the solutions according to local disposal procedures.
    b. Empty the solutions into the sink and rinse with warm water and soap.
    c. Ensure the solutions are secured in closed containers and throw away.
    d. Store the solutions in a secured, dry place for later use.

37. The volume of water in a bucket is 2.5 liters. When an object with an irregular shape and a mass of 40 grams is submerged in the water, the volume of the water is 4.5 liters. What is the density of the object?

    a. $\frac{1}{10}$ g/L
    b. 2 g/L
    c. 20 g/L
    d. 80 g/L

38. Which of the following represents a chemical change?

    a. Sublimation of water
    b. A spoiling apple
    c. Dissolution of salt in water
    d. Pulverized rock

39. The amount of potential energy an object has depends on all of the following except its:

    a. mass
    b. height above ground
    c. gravitational attraction
    d. temperature.

40. Elements on the periodic table are arranged into groups and periods and ordered according to:

    a. atomic number
    b. number of protons
    c. reactivity
    d. All of the above

41. The specific heat capacity of ice is half as much as that of liquid water. What is the result of this?

    a. It takes half the amount of energy to increase the temperature of a 1 kg sample of ice by 1°C than a 1 kg sample of water.
    b. It takes twice the amount of energy to increase the temperature of a 1 kg sample of ice by 1°C than a 1 kg sample of water.
    c. It takes a quarter the amount of energy to increase the temperature of a 1 kg sample of ice by 1°C than a 1 kg sample of water.
    d. It takes the same amount of energy to increase the temperature of a 1 kg sample of ice and a 1 kg sample of water by 1°C.

42. What happens to the temperature of a substance as it is changing phase from a liquid to a solid?

    a. Its temperature increases due to the absorption of latent heat.
    b. Its temperature decreases due to the heat of vaporization.
    c. Its temperature decreases due to the latent heat of fusion.
    d. Its temperature remains the same due to the latent heat of fusion.

43. A long nail is heated at one end. After a few seconds, the other end of the nail becomes equally hot. What type of heat transfer does this represent?

    a. Radiation
    b. Conduction
    c. Convection
    d. Entropy

44. Which of the following statements about heat transfer is not true?

    a. As the energy of a system changes, its thermal energy must change or work must be done.
    b. Heat transfer from a warmer object to a cooler object can occur spontaneously.
    c. Heat transfer can never occur from a cooler object to a warmer object.
    d. If two objects reach the same temperature, energy is no longer available for work.

45. The measure of energy within a system is called _____.

    a. temperature
    b. heat
    c. entropy
    d. thermodynamics

46. Which of the following is true of an isotope?

    a. It has a different number of protons than its element.
    b. It has a different number of electrons than its element.
    c. It has a different charge as compared to its element.
    d. It has a different number of neutrons than its element.

47. If an atom's outer shell is filled, what must be true?

    a. It reacts with other atoms through chemical reactions.
    b. It exchanges electrons to form bonds with other atoms.
    c. It has 32 electrons in its outer shell.
    d. It is a stable atom.

48. Which type of nuclear process features atomic nuclei splitting apart to form smaller nuclei?
    a. Fission
    b. Fusion
    c. Decay
    d. Ionization

49. Electrons with greater amounts of energy are found _____ the nucleus than electrons with less energy.

    a. closer to
    b. farther from
    c. more often inside
    d. more randomly around

50. The process whereby a radioactive element releases energy slowly over a long period of time to lower its energy and become more stable is best described as _____.

    a. combustion
    b. fission
    c. fusion
    d. decay

51. Which of the following is a type of simple machine?

    a. A bicycle
    b. A pair of scissors
    c. A screw
    d. A shovel

52. In which of the following scenarios is work not applied to the object?

    a. Mario moves a book from the floor to the top shelf.
    b. A book drops off the shelf and falls to the floor.
    c. Mario pushes a box of books across the room.
    d. Mario balances a book on his head and walks across the room.

53. A ball is resting on the front end of a boat. The boat is moving straight forwards toward a dock. According to Newton's first law of motion, when the front of the boat hits the dock, how will the ball's motion change?

    a. The ball will remain at rest.
    b. The ball will move backwards.
    c. The ball will move forwards.
    d. The ball will move sideways.

54. What two things are required for circular motion to occur?

    a. Acceleration and centripetal force
    b. Acceleration and gravitational force
    c. Constant speed and centripetal force
    d. Constant speed and gravitational force

55. According to Bernoulli's Principle, where will a gas flowing through a pipe exert the least amount of pressure?

    a. Where the pipe is widest
    b. Where the pipe is narrowest
    c. Where its velocity is lowest
    d. Where its kinetic energy is lowest

56. If a glass rod is rubbed with a cloth made of polyester, what will the resulting charge be on each material?

    a. The charge on the glass rod is positive and the charge on the cloth is negative.
    b. The charge on the glass rod is negative and the charge on the cloth is positive.
    c. The charge on the glass rod is neutral and the charge on the cloth is positive.
    d. The charge on the glass rod and the cloth both become neutral.

57. According to Ohm's Law, how are voltage and current related in an electrical circuit?

    a. Voltage and current are inversely proportional to one another.
    b. Voltage and current are directly proportional to one another.
    c. Voltage acts to oppose the current along an electrical circuit.
    d. Voltage acts to decrease the current along an electrical circuit.

58. A material becomes magnetic when the individual electrons of an atom _____, allowing their magnetic fields to add together.

    a. spin in pairs in opposite directions
    b. spin in pairs in the same direction
    c. spin unpaired
    d. stop spinning

59. In a parallel circuit, there are three paths: A, B and C. Path A has a resistance of 10 ohms, path B a resistance of 5 ohms and part C a resistance of 2 ohms. How do the voltage and current change for each path?

    a. Voltage and current are kept the same in each path.
    b. Voltage is greatest in path A and current is greatest in path C.
    c. Voltage is lowest in path C and current is greatest in path C.
    d. Voltage is the same for each path and current is greatest in path C.

60. A rock concert is taking place outdoors. In which of the following conditions will their sound travel the farthest?

    a. High temperature and low humidity
    b. High temperature and humidity
    c. Low temperature and humidity
    d. Low temperature and high humidity

Answer Key and Explanations

Academic Aptitude

Verbal

1. A: Expand means get bigger. Contract, shrink, diminish, and lessen mean get smaller.

2. B: Adore means love. Abhor, despise, hate, and deplore mean the opposite.

3. C: Original means new or unfamiliar, the opposite of trite, cliché, overused, and commonplace.

4. D: To cooperate is to agree or get along; to bicker, argue, quarrel, or disagree are opposites.

5. E: Pandemonium, chaos, excitement, and disarray are wild, disordered states; harmony is not.

6. B: Gleeful means joyful, delighted, and happy. Somber, serious, sad, and gloomy are opposites.

7. C: Apprehension, trepidation, dread, and anxiety are worried states; optimism or hope is not.

8. D: Dismal, dreary, bleak, and depressing are synonyms; cheery is their antonym/opposite.

9. A: Fortunate means lucky. Hapless, unlucky, tragic, and doomed all mean the opposite.

10. C: To disperse is to thin (out), dissipate, or scatter; to collect is to gather/come together.

11. C: Aware is knowledgeable/informed; oblivious, clueless, heedless, and ignorant are opposites.

12. D: Distraught means very anxious, alarmed, agitated, or distracted; tranquil is peaceful, an antonym.

13. E: Bedlam, confusion, havoc, and uproar are like disorganization/disorder; order is the opposite.

14. B: Clear means easily understood. The other choices are all antonyms.

15. A: Invite is to ask or encourage; avert means to prevent; evade and elude mean to escape.

16. A: Unique is unusual/singular/one-of-a-kind; mundane, pedestrian, and quotidian mean ordinary.

17. C: Perpetual is always, constant, ceaseless, running, or continual; occasional is once in a while.

18. B: Vexing is irritating, annoying, or aggravating. Gratifying means pleasing, the opposite.

19. D: Sagacious means wise, knowing, or astute. Ignorant means unknowing, the opposite.

20. E: Audacious means bold, brash, forward, or rude. Humble is a near opposite, meaning modest.

21. A: Deriding is mocking or scorning. Approving, praising, favoring, and commending are antonyms.

22. E: Stealthy is sneaky, secretive, sly, or furtive; transparent is open, clear, or obvious, the opposite.

23. C: Impudent means sassy, rude, impertinent, or disrespectful; respectful means the opposite.

24. D: Blissful, blithe, jubilant, and jocund mean delighted/joyful/happy; aggrieved means sad/unhappy.

25. B: Gaunt means haggard, wasted, or skinny. Plump means chubby, fat, or fleshy, the opposite.

26. A: Unassuming is modest/humble; haughty, superior, lofty, and presumptuous are proud/arrogant.

27. B: Reverent is religious; blasphemous, profane, impious, and sacrilegious are disrespecting religion.

28. C: A heretic, renegade, defector, or dissident opposes accepted beliefs; believers do not.

29. B: Cynical means mistrustful, skeptical, suspicious, negative, or pessimistic; trusting is the opposite.

30. D: Agape means openmouthed, anticipating eagerly, or agog; unmoved has the opposite meaning.

Arithmetic

1. D: This is a simple addition problem. Start with the ones column (on the right). Add the figures 6+1, 3+0, 2+3 to get the answer 537.

2. C: This is a simple addition problem with carrying. Start with the ones column and add 7+4, write down the 1 and add the 1 to the digits in the tens column. Now add 0+6+1. Write down the 7. Now add 3+8 and write down the 1. Add the 1 to the thousands column. Add 4+1+1 and write the 6 to get the answer 6171.

3. B: Simply substitute the given values for *a* and *b* and perform the required operations.

4. A: This is a subtraction problem which involves borrowing. Start with the ones column. Since 7 can't be subtracted from 6, borrow ten from the tens column. Cross out the 5 and make it a 4. Now subtract 7 from 16. Write down 9. Move to the tens column Since 6 can't be subtracted from 4, borrow ten from the hundreds column. Cross out the 3 and make it a 2.   14-6 = 8. Now subtract 1 from 2 and write down 1 to get 189.

5. B: This is a subtraction problem which also involves borrowing. Start with the ones column. Since 7 can't be subtracted from 6, borrow ten from the tens column. Cross out the 0 and make it a 9. Cross out the 2 in the hundreds column and make it a 2. Now subtract 7 from 16. Write down 9. Move to the tens column. Subtract 8 from 9 and write down 1. Move to the hundreds column. Since you can't subtract 4 from 3, borrow ten from the thousands column. Cross out the 5 and make it a 4. 12-4= 8. Now subtract 3 from 4 and write down 1 to get 1819.

6. C: This problem is solved by finding *x* in this equation: $34/80 = x/100$.

7. A: This is a multiplication problem with 0. Start with the 7 in 17 and multiply it by each of the digits at the top 7 x 7. Write down the 9 and place the 4 in the tens column. 7 x 0 is 0. Add the 4. 7 x 7 is 49. The top line will read 4949. Now multiply 1 by 7. Write down the 7. 1 x 0 is 0 and 1 x 7 is 7. The bottom line will read 707. Add these together with the 7 in the tens column and the answer will be 12,019.

- 114 -

8. A: This is a simple division problem. Divide the 7 into 9. It goes in 1 time. Write 1 above the 9 and subtract 7 from 9 to get 2. Bring down the 1 and place it beside the 2. Divide 7 into 21. It goes in 3 times. Divide 7 into 7. It goes 1 time.

9. D: To solve this problem, work backwards. That is, perform FOIL on each answer choice until you derive the original expression.

10. A: To change this fraction into a decimal, divide 100 into 38. 100 goes into 38 .38 times.

11. C: This is a simple addition problem. Line up the decimals so that they are all in the same place in the equation, and see that there is a 6 by itself in the hundredths column. Then add the tenths column: 8+3to get 11. Write down the 1 and carry the 1. Add the ones column: 6+1 plus the carried 1. Write down 8. Then write down the 1.

12. A: A set of six numbers with an average of 4 must have a collective sum of 24. The two numbers that average 2 will add up to 4, so the remaining numbers must add up to 20. The average of these four numbers can be calculated: 20/4 = 5.

13. C: Count from the 3: tenths, hundredths, thousandths.

14. A: This is a simple subtraction problem with decimals. Line up the decimals and subtract 9 from 8. Since this can't be done, borrow 10 from the 5. Cross out the 5 and make it 4. Now subtract 9 from 18 to get 9. Subtract 3 from 4 and get 1. Place the decimal point before the 1.

15. D: Simple Multiplication.

16. A: To add fractions, ensure that the denominator (the number on the bottom) is the same. Since it is not, change them both to 56ths. 1/8 equals 7/56. 3/7 equals 24/56. Now add the whole numbers: 3+6 = 9 and the fractions 31/56.

17. C: To subtract fractions, ensure that the denominator (the number on the bottom) is the same. Since it is not, change them both to 14ths. 1/7 = 2/14; 1/2 = 7/14. The equation now looks like this: $4\frac{2}{14} - 2\frac{7}{14}$. Change the 4 to 3 and add 14 to the numerator (the top number) so that the fractions can be subtracted. The equation now looks like this: $3\frac{16}{14} - 2\frac{7}{14}$. Subtract: $1\frac{9}{14}$

18. A: To multiply mixed numbers, first create improper fractions. Multiply the whole number by the denominator, then add the numerator. $1\frac{1}{4}$ becomes $\frac{5}{4}$; $3\frac{2}{5}$ becomes $\frac{17}{5}$; $1\frac{2}{3}$ becomes $\frac{5}{3}$.

The problem will look like this: $\frac{5}{4} \times \frac{17}{5} \times \frac{5}{3} = \frac{425}{60} = 7\frac{5}{60} = 7\frac{1}{12}$.

19. C: There are 12 inches in a foot and 3 feet in a yard. Four and a half yards is equal to 162 inches. To determine the number of 3-inch segments, divide 162 by 3.

20. C: Divide the numerator and denominator by 14.

21. A: Write .36, and then move the decimal two places. Add the percent sign.

22. C: 10% of 900 are 90. Multiply 90 by 4 to find 40%.

23. A: If it takes 3 people 3 1/3 days to do the job, then it would take one person 10 days: $3 \times 3\frac{1}{3} = 10$. Thus, it would take 2 people 5 days, and one day of work for two people would complete 1/5 of the job.

24. A: Divide 40 by 8 to get 5. Multiply 5 by 3 to get 15.

25. B: Rewrite the problem as 0.06*25 and solve.

26. D: Divide 4 by 16 (not 16 by 4)

27. C: Since 4 is the same as 2^2, $4^6 = 2^{12}$. When dividing exponents with the same base, simply subtract the exponent in the denominator from the exponent in the numerator.

28. D: To solve, rewrite the percent as a fraction: $\frac{30}{100}$. Then reduce the fraction.

29. C: To change a percent to a decimal, remove the percent sign and move the decimal two spaces to the left.

30. A: To solve, add 6 *a* and 2*a*, then subtract 4*a*.

Nonverbal

1. A: The first figure has a circle inside the rectangle; in the second figure, the inner shape is removed. The third figure is a circle with a rectangular inner shape. (A) is a circle like the third figure, with the inner shape removed as it is in the second figure.

2. B: The first figure is a larger rectangle, and the second figure is a smaller rectangle. The third figure is a larger circle, and (B) is a smaller circle.

3. C: The first figure is a circle with a smaller circle inside; the second figure is a rectangle with a smaller rectangle inside. The third figure is like the smaller inner circle from the first figure without the larger outer circle, and (C) is like the smaller rectangle from the second figure without the larger outer rectangle.

4. D: The first figure is a rectangle, and the second, a triangle, is one half diagonally of the first rectangle. The third figure is a circle, and (D) is one half diagonally of the circle.

5. E: Of the choices given, the corner section (E) of the rectangle in the third figure is most like the semicircular section shown in the second figure of the ring/circle shown in the first figure.

6. D: The triangle in the first figure is inverted (turned upside down) in the second figure. The semicircular shape in the third figure is also inverted in (D).

7. C: The first figure is a star with 4 points and the second figure is a star with 5 points. The third figure is a star with 6 points. Continuing the pattern of adding 1 point, (C) is a star with 7 points.

8. B: The first figure is the right half of a circle, and the second figure is a full circle. The third figure is the right half of a diamond, and (B) is a full diamond.

9. A: The first two figures are both rectangles; the first contains vertical stripes, and the second contains horizontal stripes. The third figure is a circle containing vertical stripes. Therefore, the circle containing horizontal stripes in (A) repeats the pattern.

- 116 -

10. B: The first diamond is clear, and the second is filled with a diamond-checked design. The third figure, a circle, is clear like the first diamond; therefore, the circle filled with the diamond-checked design in (B) follows the pattern.

11. C: The first figure is a small sunburst; the second figure is a larger sunburst. The third figure is a small smiley face, so the larger smiley face in (C) creates a matching relationship.

12. D: The first figure is a right-angled shape with an arrow point on one end; the second figure is a right-angled shape with arrow points on both ends. The third figure is a straight shape with an arrow point on one end, so the straight shape with arrow points on both ends (D) matches the relationship.

13. C: The first figure is like a block equal sign with a diagonal slash; the second figure is a ring/circle, also with a diagonal slash. The third figure is like the first equal sign, but with no slash. Therefore the ring with no slash (C) is most like the third figure.

14. D: The first figure is a circle filled with a checkerboard design, and the second circle is clear. The third figure is a rectangle filled with the checkerboard design, so the clear rectangle (D) corresponds.

15. E: In the first figure, two triangles are joined point to point; in the second, two hearts are joined, also point to point. In the third figure, the triangles are joined at their broader bases rather than their points; the two hearts in (E) are also joined at their broader tops rather than their points.

16. B: The first figure is a curve with an arrow pointing up; the second is a curve with an arrow pointing down. The third figure is straight with an arrow pointing up; therefore, the straight figure with an arrow pointing down (B) matches the relationship.

17. A: The first figure is a triangle filled with a zigzag design; the second is a triangle filled with a grid design. The third figure is a circle filled with a zigzag design; therefore, the circle filled with a grid design (A) shows the same relationship.

18. E: The heart in the first figure is inverted in the second figure. The third figure is a triangle; this shape is inverted in (E) the same way that the heart is.

19. E: The first figure has two crescent shapes with their points facing each other; in the second figure, the points face away. The third figure has a pair of angular brackets, facing each other like the first pair of crescents. Therefore, the pair of angular brackets facing away from each other (E) matches the second pair of crescents.

20. B: The first figure, a circle, has been elongated and narrowed into a long, thin oval in the second figure. The third figure, a diamond, is likewise made longer and thinner in (B).

21. A: The first diamond has diagonal stripes going from the lower left to the upper right; the second diamond has diagonal stripes going from the upper left to the lower right. The third figure is a circle with diagonal stripes matching those in the first diamond; therefore, the circle with diagonal stripes matching those in the second diamond follows the pattern.

22. C: The first two figures point to the right, and they would dovetail if put together. The third figure also points to the right but is rounded rather than angled; the rounded shape, also pointing right in (C), would also dovetail with the third figure if they were put together.

23. E: The first two lines have the same right angles, but the first one has arrows at both ends, pointing up and down; the second has an arrow on only one end, pointing down. The third figure is straight, with arrows at both ends. Therefore, the straight figure with an arrow on only one end pointing down (E) relates to the third figure the same way.

24. D: The first line has two right-angled bends, with one arrow at the top; the second line has the same angles, but it has arrows at both top and bottom. The third figure is curved, with one arrow at the top, so the curved line with arrows at both top and bottom (D) follows the same relationship.

25. D: The first figure has four arrow points, and the second has three. The third figure also has three arrow points. The figure with two arrow points (D) continues the pattern of subtracting one arrow point. (4 : 3 is as 3 : 2.)

26. C: The first figure is a circle with two progressively smaller circles inside. The second figure is like the first but with the smallest circle removed. The third figure is a rectangle with two progressively smaller rectangles inside, so the rectangle missing the smallest inner rectangle (C) repeats the pattern.

27. B: The first figure is a diamond with a smaller diamond inside. The second figure is like the first, but with a third, even smaller diamond inside of the others. The third figure is a circle with a smaller circle inside. Therefore, the circle containing two smaller circles (B) follows the same relationship.

28. E: The second figure, a crescent, is a section of the first figure, a circle. The third figure is a rectangle, and the corner piece (E) is correspondingly a section of it.

29. A: The second shape is the first shape, inverted. The third shape is also inverted in choice (A).

30. A: The first shape is the top half of the second shape. Likewise, the third shape is the top half of the shape in (A).

Spelling

1. A: separate

2. B: nuclear

3. C: familiar

4. A: sacrilegious

5. C: agitated

6. B: oriented

7. C: indispensable

8. A: similar

9. B: attitude

10. B: abbreviate

11. A: absorb

12. C: accumulate

13. C: aerial

14. A: comedian

15. B: asphalt

16. B: forcible

17. C: anecdote

18. A: flexible

19. A: defendant

20. C: plaintiff

21. B: idiosyncrasy

22. A: hazardous

23. B: horrific

24. C: handsome

25. A: liaison

26. B: galaxy

27. A: attorneys

28. C: asterisk

29. C: equilibrium

30. A: brilliance

31. B: blanch.

32. A: ecstasy

33. B: depreciate

34. C: turpitude

35. B: opposite

36. C: tyranny

37. A: schism

38. C: schedule

39. A: incandescent

40. B: terrific

41. B: homogenize

42. A: sieve

43. C: truly

44. A: sincerely

45. B: transient

46. A: sedition

47. C: thieves

48. B: vengeance

49. B: nylon

50. C: unacceptable

51. A: deficit

52. B: disapproval

53. A: diffidence

54. C: picnicking

55. C: oregano

56. B: bachelor

57. A: indelible

58. B: diurnal

59. A: impatience

60. C: parliament

Natural Science

1. D: The name for a substance that stimulates the production of antibodies is an *antigen*. An antigen is any substance perceived by the immune system as dangerous. When the body senses an antigen, it produces an antibody. *Collagen* is one of the components of bone, tendon, and cartilage. It is a spongy protein that can be turned into gelatin by boiling. *Hemoglobin* is the part of red blood cells that carries oxygen. In order for the blood to carry enough oxygen to the cells of the body, there has to be a sufficient amount of hemoglobin. *Lymph* is a near-transparent fluid that performs a number of functions in the body: It removes bacteria from tissues, replaces lymphocytes in the blood, and moves fat away from the small intestine. Lymph contains white blood cells. As you can see, some of the questions in the vocabulary section will require technical knowledge.

2. D: The cellular hierarchy starts with the cell, the simplest structure, and progresses to organisms, the most complex structures.

3. B: A hypertonic solution is a solution with a higher particle concentration than in the cell, and consequently lower water content than in the cell. Water moves from the cell to the solution, causing the cell to experience water loss and shrink.

4. A: The immune system consists of the lymphatic system, spleen, tonsils, thymus and bone marrow.

5. D: The rate at which a chemical reaction occurs does not depend on the amount of mass lost, since the law of conservation of mass (or matter) states that in a chemical reaction there is no loss of mass.

6. B: Boyle's law states that for a constant mass and temperature, pressure and volume are related inversely to one another: $PV = c$, where c = constant.

7. C: Prokaryotic cells are simpler cells that do not have membrane-bound organelles, whereas eukaryotic cells have several membrane-bound organelles.

8. A: A ribosome is a structure of eukaryotic cells that makes proteins.

9. B: It is impossible for an *AaBb* organism to have the *aa* combination in the gametes. It is impossible for each letter to be used more than one time, so it would be impossible for the lowercase *a* to appear twice in the gametes. It would be possible, however, for *Aa* to appear in the gametes, since there is one uppercase *A* and one lowercase *a*. Gametes are the cells involved in sexual reproduction. They are germ cells.

10. B: The oxidation number of the hydrogen in CaH_2 is -1. The oxidation number is the positive or negative charge of a monoatomic ion. In other words, the oxidation number is the numerical charge on an ion. An ion is a charged version of an element. Oxidation number is often referred to as oxidation state. Oxidation number is sometimes used to describe the number of electrons that must be added or removed from an atom in order to convert the atom to its elemental form.

11. C: *Prolactin* stimulates the production of breast milk during lactation. *Norepinephrine* is a hormone and neurotransmitter secreted by the adrenal gland that regulates heart rate, blood pressure, and blood sugar. *Antidiuretic hormone* is produced by the hypothalamus and secreted by the pituitary gland. It regulates the concentration of urine and triggers the contractions of the arteries and capillaries. *Oxytocin* is a hormone secreted by the pituitary gland that makes it easier to eject milk from the breast and manages the contractions of the uterus during labor.

12. A: The typical result of mitosis in humans is two diploid cells. *Mitosis* is the division of a body cell into two daughter cells. Each of the two produced cells has the same set of chromosomes as the parent. A diploid cell contains both sets of homologous chromosomes. A haploid cell contains only one set of chromosomes, which means that it only has a single set of genes.

13. A: Boron does not exist as a diatomic molecule. The other possible answer choices, fluorine, oxygen, and nitrogen, all exist as diatomic molecules. A diatomic molecule always appears in nature as a pair: The word *diatomic* means "having two atoms." With the exception of astatine, all of the halogens are diatomic. Chemistry students often use the mnemonic BrINClHOF (pronounced "brinkelhoff") to remember all of the diatomic elements: bromine, iodine, nitrogen, chlorine, hydrogen, oxygen, and fluorine. Note that not all of these diatomic elements are halogens.

14. D: Of the given structures, veins have the lowest blood pressure. *Veins* carry oxygen-poor blood from the outlying parts of the body to the heart. An *artery* carries oxygen-rich blood from the heart to the peripheral parts of the body. An *arteriole* extends from an artery to a capillary. A *venule* is a tiny vein that extends from a capillary to a larger vein.

15. B: Water stabilizes the temperature of living things. The ability of warm-blooded animals, including human beings, to maintain a constant internal temperature is known as *homeostasis*. Homeostasis depends on the presence of water in the body. Water tends to minimize changes in temperature because it takes a while to heat up or cool down. When the human body gets warm, the blood vessels dilate and blood moves away from the torso and toward the extremities. When the body gets cold, blood concentrates in the torso. This is the reason why hands and feet tend to get especially cold in cold weather.

16. D: Hydriodic acid is another name for aqueous HI. In an aqueous solution, the solvent is water. Hydriodic acid is a polyatomic ion, meaning that it is composed of two or more elements. When this solution has an increased amount of oxygen, the *-ate* suffix on the first word is converted to *-ic*.

17. C: Of the four heart chambers, the left ventricle is the most muscular. When it contracts, it pushes blood out to the organs and extremities of the body. The right ventricle pushes blood into the lungs. The atria, on the other hand, receive blood from the outlying parts of the body and transport it into the ventricles. The basic process works as follows: Oxygen-poor blood fills the right atrium and is pumped into the right ventricle, from which it is pumped into the pulmonary artery and on to the lungs. In the lungs, this blood is oxygenated. The blood then reenters the heart at the left atrium, which when full pumps into the left ventricle. When the left ventricle is full, blood is pushed into the aorta and on to the organs and extremities of the body.

18. B: Oxygen is not one of the products of the Krebs cycle. The *Krebs cycle* is the second stage of cellular respiration. In this stage, a sequence of reactions converts pyruvic acid into carbon dioxide. This stage of cellular respiration produces the phosphate compounds that provide most of the energy for the cell. The Krebs cycle is also known as the citric acid cycle or the tricarboxylic acid cycle.

19. A: A limiting reactant is entirely used up by the chemical reaction. Limiting reactants control the extent of the reaction and determine the quantity of the product. A reducing agent is a substance that reduces the amount of another substance by losing electrons. A reagent is any substance used in a chemical reaction. Some of the most common reagents in the laboratory are sodium hydroxide and hydrochloric acid. The behavior and properties of these substances are known, so they can be effectively used to produce predictable reactions in an experiment.

20. A: The *cerebrum* is the part of the brain that interprets sensory information. It is the largest part of the brain. The cerebrum is divided into two hemispheres, connected by a thin band of tissue called the corpus callosum. The *cerebellum* is positioned at the back of the head, between the brain stem and the cerebrum. It controls both voluntary and involuntary movements. The *medulla oblongata* forms the base of the brain. This part of the brain is responsible for blood flow and breathing, among other things.

21. C: The sugar and phosphate in DNA are connected by covalent bonds. A *covalent bond* is formed when atoms share electrons. It is very common for atoms to share pairs of electrons. An *ionic bond* is created when one or more electrons are transferred between atoms. *Ionic bonds*, also known as *electrovalent bonds*, are formed between ions with opposite charges. There is no such thing as an *overt bond* in chemistry.

22. C: The mass of 7.35 mol water is 132 grams. You should be able to find the mass of various chemical compounds when you are given the number of mols. The information required to perform this function is included on the periodic table. To solve this problem, find the molecular mass of water by finding the respective weights of hydrogen and oxygen. Remember that water contains two hydrogen molecules and one oxygen molecule. The molecular mass of hydrogen is roughly 1, and the molecular mass of oxygen is roughly 16. A molecule of water, then, has approximately 18 grams of mass. Multiply this by 7.35 mol, and you will obtain the answer 132.3, which is closest to answer choice C.

23. C: *Collagen* is the protein produced by cartilage. Bone, tendon, and cartilage are all mainly composed of collagen. *Actin* and *myosin* are the proteins responsible for muscle contractions. Actin makes up the thinner fibers in muscle tissue, while myosin makes up the thicker fibers. Myosin is the most numerous cell protein in human muscle. *Estrogen* is one of the steroid hormones produced mainly by the ovaries. Estrogen motivates the menstrual cycle and the development of female sex characteristics.

24. B: Unlike other organic molecules, lipids are not water soluble. Lipids are typically composed of carbon and hydrogen. Three common types of lipid are fats, waxes, and oils. Indeed, lipids usually feel oily when you touch them. All living cells are primarily composed of lipids, carbohydrates, and proteins. Some examples of fats are lard, corn oil, and butter. Some examples of waxes are beeswax and carnauba wax. Some examples of steroids are cholesterol and ergosterol.

25. D: Of these orbitals, the last to fill is 6s. Orbitals fill in the following order: 1s, 2s, 2p, 3s, 3p, 4s, 3d, 4p, 5s, 4d, 5p, 6s, 4f, 5d, 6p, 7s, 5f, 6d, and 7p. The number is the orbital number, and the letter is the sublevel identification. Sublevel s has one orbital and can hold a maximum of two electrons. Sublevel p has three orbitals and can hold a maximum of six electrons. Sublevel d has five orbitals and can hold a maximum of 10 electrons. Sublevel f has seven orbitals and can hold a maximum of 14 electrons.

26. C: The parasympathetic nervous system is responsible for lowering the heart rate. It slows down the heart rate, dilates the blood vessels, and increases the secretions of the digestive system. The central nervous system is composed of the brain and the spinal cord. The sympathetic nervous system is a part of the autonomic nervous system; its role is to oppose the actions taken by the parasympathetic nervous system. So, the sympathetic nervous system accelerates the heart, contracts the blood vessels, and decreases the secretions of the digestive system.

27. D: *Hemoglobin* is not a steroid. It is a protein that helps to move oxygen from the lungs to the various body tissues. Steroids can be either synthetic chemicals used to reduce swelling and

inflammation or sex hormones produced by the body. *Cholesterol* is the most abundant steroid in the human body. It is necessary for the creation of bile, though it can be dangerous if the levels in the body become too high. *Estrogen* is a female steroid produced by the ovaries (in females), testes (in males), placenta, and adrenal cortex. It contributes to adolescent sexual development, menstruation, mood, lactation, and aging. *Testosterone* is the main hormone produced by the testes; it is responsible for the development of adult male sex characteristics.

28. C: Nitrogen pentoxide is the name of the binary molecular compound NO_5. The format given in answer choice C is appropriate when dealing with two nonmetals. A prefix is used to denote the number of atoms of each element. Note that when there are seven atoms of a given element, the prefix *hepta-* is used instead of the usual *septa-*. Also, when the first atom in this kind of binary molecular compound is single, it does not need to be given the prefix *mono-*.

29. B: Smooth muscle tissue is said to be arranged in a disorderly fashion because it is not striated like the other two types of muscle: cardiac and skeletal. Striations are lines that can only be seen with a microscope. *Smooth* muscle is typically found in the supporting tissues of hollow organs and blood vessels. *Cardiac* muscle is found exclusively in the heart; it is responsible for the contractions that pump blood throughout the body. *Skeletal* muscle, by far the most preponderant in the body, controls the movements of the skeleton. The contractions of skeletal muscle are responsible for all voluntary motion. There is no such thing as *rough* muscle.

30. C: *Melatonin* is produced by the pineal gland. One of the primary functions of melatonin is regulation of the circadian cycle, which is the rhythm of sleep and wakefulness. *Insulin* helps regulate the amount of glucose in the blood. Without insulin, the body is unable to convert blood sugar into energy. *Testosterone* is the main hormone produced by the testes; it is responsible for the development of adult male sex characteristics. *Epinephrine*, also known as adrenaline, performs a number of functions: It quickens and strengthens the heartbeat and dilates the bronchioles. Epinephrine is one of the hormones secreted when the body senses danger.

31. B: 0.05. In the metric system, 5 decimeters is equal to 0.05 decameters. A meter is the standard measurement of length. Prefixes are defined in increments of 10 to increase or decrease quantity. The prefix "deci" is equivalent to 10-1 or a tenth (0.1). A decimeter would be equal to 0.1 meters. The prefix "deca" is equivalent to 10 or 101. A decameter would be equal to 10 meters. To convert a smaller unit to a larger one, move the decimal place to the left. Since 10 decimeters make up 1 meter, for 5 decimeters, move the decimal 1 place to the left to find meters, which would be 0.5 meters. Because a decameter is larger than 1 meter (10 meters in 1 decameter), move the decimal another place to the left to change from meters to decameters, which would be 0.05 decameters. An alternate method is to set up conversion factors. This method involves canceling units and is very helpful to learn for other scientific problems.

32. C: The distribution of weight among players of a football team. In this case, a pie chart can illustrate the whole number of players as well as the number (or percentage) of players at given weights. It would be easy to interpret the data that, for example, 75% of the team weigh 250 pounds or more, 20% weigh between 200 and 250 pounds, and a mere 5% weight less than 200 pounds. The other answers would be better served in bar or line charts to compare variables or amounts that do not vary greatly.

33. D: Electrophoresis. Electrophoresis, also known as gel electrophoresis, uses electrical charges to separate substances such as protein, DNA and RNA. Depending upon the electrical charge and size of the molecules, they will travel through a porous gel at different rates when a charge is applied. Answer A, Spectrophotometry, refers to the measurement of visible light, near-ultraviolet, and

near-infrared wavelengths. Answer B, Chromatography, refers to a number of techniques that separate mixtures of chemicals based on the differences in the compound's affinity for a stationary phase, usually a porous solid, and a mobile phase, which can be either a liquid or a gas. Answer C, Centrifugation, separates mixtures by spinning to generate centripetal force, which causes heavier particles to separate from lighter particles.

34. A: By multiplying the ocular lens power times the objective being used. When using a light microscope, total magnification is determined by multiplying the ocular lens power times the objective being used. The ocular lens refers to the eyepiece, which has one magnification strength, typically 10x. The objective lens also has a magnification strength, often 4x, 10x, 40x or 100x. Using a 10x eyepiece with the 4x objective lens will give a magnification strength of 40x. Using a 10x eyepiece with the 100x objective lens will give a magnification strength of 1,000x. The shorter lens is the lesser magnification; the longer lens is the greater magnification.

35. C: Decaying specimens are never permitted but unknown specimens are sometimes permitted. When performing a dissection in class, decaying specimens can be permitted but unknown specimens are never permitted. Answer A, Rinse the specimen before handling, can help wash away excess preservative, which may be irritating. Answer B, Dispose of harmful chemicals according to district regulations; this is always required. Answer D, Students with open sores on their hands that cannot be covered should be excused from the dissection, is a good precaution. Exposure to pathogens and toxic chemicals can occur through open breaks in the skin.

36. A: Dispose of the solutions according to local disposal procedures. Solutions and compounds used in labs may be hazardous according to state and local regulatory agencies and should be treated with such precaution. Answer B, Empty the solutions into the sink and rinse with warm water and soap, does not take into account the hazards associated with a specific solution in terms of vapors, or interactions with water, soap and waste piping systems. Answer C, Ensure the solutions are secured in closed containers and throw away, may allow toxic chemicals to get into landfills and subsequently into fresh water systems. Answer D, Store the solutions in a secured, dry place for later use, is incorrect as chemicals should not be re-used due to the possibility of contamination.

37. C: 20 g/L. One way to measure the density of an irregularly shaped object is to submerge it in water and measure the displacement. This is done by taking the mass (40 grams), then finding the volume by measuring how much water it displaces. Fill a graduated cylinder with water and record the amount. Put the object in the water and record the water level. Subtract the difference in water levels to get the amount of water displaced, which is also the volume of the object. In this case, 4.5 liters minus 2.5 liters equals 2 liters. Divide mass by volume (40 grams divided by 2 liters) to get 20 g/L (grams per liter).

38. B: A spoiling apple. A spoiling apple is an example of a chemical change. During a chemical change, one substance is changed into another. Oxidation, a chemical change, occurs when an apple spoils. Answer A, Sublimation of water, refers to the conversion between the solid and the gaseous phases of matter, with no intermediate liquid stage. This is a phase change, not a chemical reaction. Answer C, Dissolution of salt in water, refers to a physical change, since the salt and water can be separated again by evaporating the water, which is a physical change. Answer D, Pulverized rock, is an example of a physical change where the form has changed but not the substance itself.

39. D: The amount of potential energy an object has depends on mass, height above ground and gravitational attraction, but not temperature. The formula for potential energy is PE = mgh, or potential energy equals mass times gravity times height. Answers A, B, and C are all valid answers

as they are all contained in the formula for potential energy. Potential energy is the amount of energy stored in a system particularly because of its position.

40. D: Elements on the periodic table are arranged into periods, or rows, according to atomic number, which is the number of protons in the nucleus. The periodic table illustrates the recurrence of properties. Each column, or group, contains elements that share similar properties, such as reactivity.

41. A: It takes half the amount of energy to increase the temperature of a 1 kg sample of ice by 1°C than a 1 kg sample of water. Heat capacity refers to the amount of heat or thermal energy required to raise the temperature of a specific substance a given unit. A substance with a higher heat capacity requires more heat to raise its temperature than a substance with a lower heat capacity. The comparison here is that the specific heat capacity of ice is half as much as that of liquid water, so it takes half the amount of energy to increase the same amount of ice one temperature unit than it would if it were liquid water.

42. D: Its temperature remains the same due to the latent heat of fusion. The temperature of a substance during the time of any phase change remains the same. In this case, the phase change was from liquid to solid, or freezing. Latent heat of fusion, in this case, is energy that is released from the substance as it reforms its solid form. This energy will be released and the liquid will turn to solid before the temperature of the substance will decrease further. If the substance were changing from solid to liquid, the heat of fusion would be the amount of heat required to break apart the attractions between the molecules in the solid form to change to the liquid form. The latent heat of fusion is exactly the same quantity of energy for a substance for either melting or freezing. Depending on the process, this amount of heat would either be absorbed by the substance (melting) or released (freezing).

43. B: A long nail or other type of metal, substance or matter that is heated at one end and then the other end becomes equally hot is an example of conduction. Conduction is energy transfer by neighboring molecules from an area of hotter temperature to cooler temperature. Answer A, Radiation, or thermal radiation, refers to heat being transferred through empty space by electromagnetic radiation. An example is sunlight heating the earth. Answer C, Convection, refers to heat being transferred by molecules moving from one location in the substance to another creating a heat current, usually in a gas or a liquid. Answer D, Entropy, relates to the second law of thermodynamics and refers to how much heat or energy is no longer available to do work in a system. It can also be stated as the amount of disorder in a system.

44. C: Heat transfer can never occur from a cooler object to a warmer object. While the second law of thermodynamics implies that heat never spontaneously transfers from a cooler object to a warmer object, it is possible for heat to be transferred to a warmer object, given the proper input of work to the system. This is the principle by which a refrigerator operates. Work is done to the system to transfer heat from the objects inside the refrigerator to the air surrounding the refrigerator. All other answer choices are true.

45. B: The measure of energy within a system is called heat. Answer A, temperature, is a measurement of the average kinetic energy of molecules in a substance. A higher temperature means greater kinetic energy or faster moving molecules. Answer C, entropy, is the amount of energy that is no longer available for work, related to the second law of thermodynamics. Answer D, thermodynamics, is the study of the conversion of energy into heat and work in a system.

46. D: It has a different number of neutrons than its element. An isotope is a variation of an element that has a different number of neutrons. The element and its various isotopes continue to have the same numbers of protons and electrons. For example, carbon has three naturally occurring isotopes, carbon-12, carbon-13 and carbon-14, which is radioactive. Isotopes of an element differ in mass number, which is the number of protons and neutrons added together, but have the same atomic number, or number of protons.

47. D: It is a stable atom. If an atom's outer shell is filled, it is a stable atom. The outer shell refers to one of many energy levels, or shells, that electrons occupy around a nucleus. An atom whose outer shell is not filled wants to become stable by filling the outer shell. It fills its outer shell by forming bonds. The atom can do this by gaining electrons or losing electrons in ionic compounds, or if the atom is a part of a molecule, by sharing electrons. If an atom has a full outer shell, such as the noble gases, it does not readily react with other atoms and does not exchange electrons to form bonds. These atoms are known as inert. Therefore, Answers A and B cannot be true. Answer C, It has 32 electrons in its outer shell, is not necessarily true because not all elements have the fourth shell that can hold 32 electrons. Some have fewer shells that hold fewer electrons.

48. A: Fission is a nuclear process where atomic nuclei split apart to form smaller nuclei. Nuclear fission can release large amounts of energy, emit gamma rays and form daughter products. It is used in nuclear power plants and bombs. Answer B, Fusion, refers to a nuclear process whereby atomic nuclei join to form a heavier nucleus, such as with stars. This can release or absorb energy depending upon the original elements. Answer C, Decay, refers to an atomic nucleus spontaneously losing energy and emitting ionizing particles and radiation. Answer D, Ionization, refers to a process by which atoms obtain a positive or negative charge because the number of electrons does not equal that of protons.

49. B: Electrons with greater amounts of energy are found farther from the nucleus than electrons with less energy. The principle quantum number describes the level or shell that an electron is in. The lower the number, the closer the electron is to the nucleus and the lower it is in energy.

50. D: The process whereby a radioactive element releases energy slowly over a long period of time to lower its energy and become more stable is best described as decay. The nucleus undergoing decay, known as the parent nuclide, spontaneously releases energy most commonly through the emission of an alpha particle, a beta particle or a gamma ray. The changed nucleus, called the daughter nuclide, is now more stable than the parent nuclide, although the daughter nuclide may undergo another decay to an even more stable nucleus. A decay chain is a series of decays of a radioactive element into different more stable elements.

51. C: A screw is a type of simple machine. A screw is an inclined plane wrapped around a shaft. A wedge is also an inclined plane. A compound machine is a machine that employs two or more simple machines. Answer A, a bicycle, is a compound machine, consisting of a combination of the simple machines: wheels, levers, pulleys and wedges (used as stoppers). Answer B, a pair of scissors, is also a compound machine consisting of two wedges (the blades) that pivot on a lever. Answer D, a shovel, is a compound machine consisting of a lever (the handle) and a wedge (the head of the shovel).

52. D: Mario balances a book on his head and walks across the room. In this example, work is not applied to the book by Mario. Work is defined as a force acting on an object to cause displacement. In this case, the book was not displaced in the direction of the force applied to it. Mario's head applied a vertical force to the book. By moving horizontally across the room, the movement of the book was not in the direction of the force applied. Therefore, there was no work applied to the

- 126 -

book by Mario. In Answer A, Mario moves a book from the floor to the top shelf. Mario lifted the book vertically, in the same direction as the force applied. Therefore, work was done. In Answer B, A book drops off the shelf and falls to the floor, gravity has acted as the force and work was done. In Answer C, Mario pushes a box of books across the room, is also an example of work.

53. C: The ball will move forwards. Newton's first law of motion states that an object in motion tends to stay in motion until a force acts to change it. The ball is moving forward with the boat. When the front of the boat hits the dock, the ball's motion does not change. It continues to move forward because the force acting to stop the boat is not acting upon the ball. The forward motion of the boat is halted by the dock. The forward motion of the ball is not stopped. Since the ball is round there is little friction to provide an equal and opposite reaction to the forward motion.

54. A: Acceleration and centripetal force. Acceleration and centripetal force are required for circular motion to occur. Acceleration is defined as a change in direction of velocity. Centripetal force is toward the center, or inward force. Answer B, Acceleration and gravitational force, is incorrect because the force of gravity is not required for circular motion. Answer C, Constant speed and centripetal force, is also incorrect as constant speed is not required for circular motion to occur. Speed can vary and circular motion can still occur. Answer D, Constant speed and gravitational force is also incorrect as constant speed nor gravitational force are required for circular motion to occur.

55. B: Where the pipe is narrowest. A fluid, either a gas or a liquid, will flow faster through a narrow section of a pipe than a wider section of pipe. Bernoulli's Principle says that the faster a fluid flows, the less pressure the fluid exerts. Therefore, a fluid will exert a lower amount of pressure in the narrow section of pipe. A fluid moving through the pipe has the same flow throughout the wider and narrow portions. This means that the same volume and mass of fluid must go a specific distance in a certain amount of time. In a narrow portion of pipe, there is less area for the same volume and mass of fluid to flow, so the fluid must move faster to maintain the same flow as in the wider portion of pipe. A fluid moving faster through a narrow portion of pipe will exert less pressure and a fluid moving slower through a wide section of pipe will exert a greater pressure.

56. A: The charge on the glass rod is positive and the charge on the cloth is negative when the glass rod is rubbed with a cloth made of polyester. This is an example of static electricity — the collection of electrically charged particles on the surface of a material. A static charge can be quickly discharged, commonly called a "spark", or discharged more slowly by dissipating to the ground. A static charge occurs because different materials have a capacity for giving up electrons and becoming positive (+), or for attracting electrons and becoming negative (-). The triboelectric series is a list of materials and their propensities for either giving up electrons to become positive or to gain the electrons to become negative. Polyester has a tendency to gain electrons to become negative and glass has a tendency to lose electrons to become positive.

57. B: Voltage and current are directly proportional to one another. Ohm's Law states that voltage and current in an electrical circuit are directly proportional to one another. Ohm's Law can be expressed as $V=IR$, where V is voltage, I is current and R is resistance. Voltage is also known as electrical potential difference and is the force that moves electrons through a circuit. For a given amount of resistance, an increase in voltage will result in an increase in current. Resistance and current are inversely proportional to each other. For a given voltage, an increase in resistance will result in a decrease in current.

58. C: In an atom with paired electrons, the opposite spins of each electron in the pair cancel out the magnetic field of each electron. A material becomes magnetic when the individual electrons of an

atom spin unpaired thus allowing their magnetic fields to add together. The spin of an unpaired electron generates its own magnetic field. This can be used to make a magnet. When an external magnetic field is applied, these spins are lined up and the combined forces make a magnet.

59. D: Voltage is the same for each path and current is greatest in path C. In a parallel circuit, the voltage is the same for all three paths. Because the resistance is different on each path but the voltage is the same, Ohm's law dictates that the current will also be different for each path. Ohm's law says that current is inversely related to resistance. Therefore, the current will be greatest in path C as it has the least resistance, 2 ohms.

60. B: High temperature and humidity. Sound travels the farthest with high temperature and humidity. Sound is a mechanical wave. The sound wave travels through matter by causing a molecule to vibrate which then collides with a neighboring molecule causing it to vibrate and so on. A solid whose molecules are closely packed together will transmit the wave faster than a liquid or a gas whose particles are further apart. This is because the solid particles are more rigid and will respond to the disturbance quicker than a liquid or a gas, whose molecules are fluid. For this reason, solids can also propagate a wave further than a liquid or a gas. The principles of how sound travels through a solid can be applied to sound traveling through the air, as in this question. Air that is high in humidity has a higher density than dry air and can propagate the sound wave faster and farther than dry air. Sound waves also travel faster and farther at high temperatures. This is because at higher temperatures molecules have more kinetic energy to transmit the sound wave. At higher temperatures, molecules will also have more collisions which will result in the sound wave traveling farther and faster.

Special Report: Musculature/Innervation Review of the Arm and Back

Muscle	Origin	Insertion	Nerve
Trapezius	Ext. Occipit Protuberance, Spines of T Vertebrae	Lateral Clavicle, Spine of the Scapula	Spinal Accessory Nerve CN XI
Latissimus Dorsi	Spines of Lower 6 T Vertebrae, Iliac Crest and Lower 4 Ribs	Bicipital Groove	Thoracodorsal
Levator Scapulae	Transverse Process of C1-C4	Upper Medial Border of Scapula	Dorsal Scapula
Rhomboid Major	Spinous Process of T2-T5	Medial Border Scapula Below Spine	Dorsal Scapular
Rhomboid Minor	Spinous Process of C7-T1	Medial Border Scapula Opp. Spine	Dorsal Scapular
Teres Major	Lateral Dorsal Inferior Angle of Scapula	Bicipital Groove	Lower Subscapular
Teres Minor	Lateral Scapula 2/3 way down	Greater Tubercle of Humerus	Axillary
Deltoid	Lateral 1/3 Clavicle and Acromion Process, Spine of the Scapula	Deltoid Tuberosity	Axillary
Supraspinatus	Supraspinatus Fossa	Greater Tubercle of Humerus	Suprascapular
Infraspinatus	Infaspinatus Fossa	Greater Tubercle of Humerus	Suprascapular
Subscapularis	Subscapular Fossa	Lesser Tubercle of Humerus	Upper and lower Subscapular
Serratus Anterior	Slips of Upper 8-9 Ribs	Ventral-Medial Border Scapula	Long Thoracic
Subclavius	Inferior Surface of the Clavicle	First Rib	Nerve to the Subclavius
Pectoralis Major	Medial ½ clavicle and Side of Sternum	Bicipital Groove	Medial and Lateral Pectoral
Pectoralis Minor	Ribs 3,4,5 or 2,3,4	Coracoid Process	Medial Pectoral
Biceps Branchii	Supraglenoid Tubercle	Posterior Margin of Radial Tuberosity	Musculocutaneous
Coracobrachialis	Coracoid Process	Medial Humerus at Deltoid Tuberosity Level	Musculocutaneous
Brachialis	Anterior-Lateral ½ of Humerus	Ulnar Tuberosity and Coronoid Process	Musculocutaneous

Triceps Brachii	Infraglenoid Tubercle, Below and Medial to the Radial Groove	Olecranon Process	Radial
Anconeus	Posterior, Lateral Humeral Condyle	Upper Posterior Ulna	Radial
Brachioradialis	Lateral Supracondylar Ridge of Humerus	Radial Styloid Process	Radial
Pronator Teres	Medial Epicondyle and Supracondylar Ridge	½ Way Down on Lateral Radius	Median
Pronator Quadratus	Distal-Medial Ulna	Distal-Lateral Radius	Anterior Interosseous

Musculature/Innervation Review of the Forearm

Muscle	Origin	Insertion	Nerve
Brachioradialis	Lateral Supracondylar Ridge of Humerus	Radial Styloid Process	Radial
Pronator Teres	Medial Epicondyle and Supracondylar Ridge	½ Way Down on Lateral Radius	Median
Pronator Quadratus	Distal-Medial Ulna	Distal-Lateral Radius	Anterior Interosseous
Supinator	Lateral Epicondyle of Humerus	Upper ½ Lateral, Posterior Radius	Posterior Inter-Deep Radial
Flexor Carpi Radialis	Medial Epicondyle of Humerus	2nd and 3rd Metacarpal	Median
Flexor Carpi Ulnaris	Medial Epicondyle of Humerus	Pisiform, Hamate, 5th Metacarpal	Ulnar
Palmaris Longus	Medial Epicondyle of the Humerus	Palmar Aponeurosis and Flexor Retinaculum	Median
Flexor Digitorum Suerficialis	Medial Epicondyle, Radius, Ulna	Medial 4 Digits	Median
Flexor Digitorum Profundus	Ulna, Interosseous Membrane	Medial 4 Digits (distal part)	Median (lateral 2 digits), Ulnar (median 2 digits)
Flexor Pollicis Longus	Radius	Distal Phalanx (thumb)	Anterior Inter-Deep Median
Extensor Carpi Radialis Longus	Lateral Condyle and Supracondylar Ridge	2nd Metacarpal	Radial
Extensor Carpi Radialis Brevis	Lateral Epicondyle of Humerus	3rd Metacarpal	Posterior Inter-Deep Radial
Extensor Carpi Ulnaris	Lateral Epicondyle of Humerus	5th Metacarpal	Posterior Inter-Deep Radial
Extensor Digitorum	Lateral Epicondyle of Humerus	Extension Expansion Hood of Medial 4 Digits	Posterior Inter-Deep Radial
Extensor Digiti Minimi	Lateral Epicondyle of Humerus	Extension Expansion Hood of (little finger)	Posterior Inter-Deep Radial
Abductor Pollicis Longus	Posterior Radius and Ulna	Radial Side of 1st Metacarpal	Posterior Inter-Deep Radial
Extensor Indicis	Ulna and Interosseous Membrane	Extension Expansion Hood (index finger)	Posterior Inter-Deep Radial
Extensor Pollicis Longus	Ulna and Interosseous Membrane	Distal Phalanx (thumb)	Posterior Inter-Deep Radial
Extensor Pollicis Brevis	Radius	Proximal Phalanx (thumb)	Posterior Inter-Deep Radial

Musculature/Innervation Review of the Hand

Muscle	Origin	Insertion	Nerve
Adductor Policis	Capitate and Base of Adjacent Metacarpals	Proximal Phalanx (thumb)	Deep Branch of Ulnar
Lumbricals	Tendons of Flexor Digitorum Profundas	Extension Expansion Hood of Medial 4 Digits	Deep Branch Ulnar (medial 2 Ls), Median (lateral 2 Ls)
Dorsal Interosseous Muscles (4)	Sides of Metacarpals	Extension Expansion Hood of Digits 2-4	Deep Branch Ulnar
Palmar Interosseous (3)	Sides of Metacarpals	Extension Expansion Hood, Digits 2,4,5	Deep Branch Ulnar
Palmaris Brevis	Anterior Flexor Retinaculum and Palmar Aponeurosis	Skin-Ulnar Border of Hand	Superficial Ulnar
Abductor Pollicis Brevis	Flexor Retinaculum, Trapezium	Lateral Proximal Phalanx (thumb)	Median (thenar branch)
Flexor Pollicis Brevis	Flexor Retinaculum, Trapezium	Lateral Proximal Phalanx (thumb)	Median (thenar branch)
Opponens Pollicis	Flexor Retinaculum, Trapezium	Radial Border (1st Metacarpal)	Median (thenar branch)
Abductor Digiti Minimi	Flexor Retinaculum, Pisiform	Proximal Phalanx (little finger)	Deep Branch Ulnar
Flexor Digiti Minimi	Flexor Retinaculum, Hamate	Proximal Phalanx (little finger)	Deep Branch Ulnar
Opponens Digiti Minimi	Flexor Retinaculum, Hamate	Ulnar Medial Border (5th Metacarpal)	Deep Branch Ulnar

Musculature/Innervation Review of the Thigh

Muscle	Origin	Insertion	Nerve
Psoas Major	Bodies and Discs of T12-L5	Lesser Trochanter	L2,3
Psoas Minor	Bodies and Discs of T12 and L1	Pectineal Line of Superior Pubic Bone	L2,3
Iliacus	Upper 2/3 Iliac Fossa	Lesser Trochanter	Femoral L2-4
Pectinius	Pubic Ramus	Spiral Line	Femoral
Iliposoas	Joining of Psoas Major and Iliacus	Lesser Trochanter	L2-4
Piriformis	Anterior Surface of the Sacrum	Greater Trochanter	S1, S2
Obturator Internus	Inner Surface of the Obturator Membrane	Greater Trochanter	Sacral Plexus
Obturator Externus	Outer Surface of the Obturator Membrane	Greater Trochanter	Obturator
Gemellus Superior	Ischial Spine	Greater Trochanter	Sacral Plexus
Gemellus Inferior	Ischial Tuberosity	Greater Trochanter	Sacral Plexus
Quadratus Femoris	Ischial Tuberosity	Quadrate Tubercle of the Femur	Sacral Plexus
Gluteus Maximus	Outer Surface of Ilium, Sacrum and Coccyx	Iliotibial Tract, Gluteal Tubercle of the Femur	Inferior Gluteal
Gluteus Minimus	Outer Surface of the Ilium	Greater Trochanter	Superior Gluteal
Gluteus Medius	Outer Surface of the Ilium	Greater Trochanter	Superior Gluteal
Satorius	Anterior Superior Iliac Spine	Upper Medial Tibia	Femoral
Quadriceps Femoris	Anterior Inferior Iliac Spine, Femur-Lateral and Medial	Tibial Tuberosity	Femoral
Gracilis	Pubic Bone	Upper Medial Tibia	Obturator (anterior branch)
Abductor Longus	Pubic Bone	Linea Aspera	Obturator (anterior branch)
Abductor Brevis	Pubic Bone	Linea Aspera	Obturator (anterior branch)
Abductor Magnus	Pubic Bone	Entire Linea Aspera	Sciatic, Obturator
Tensor Faciae Latae	Iliac Crest	Iliotibial Band	Superior Gluteal
Biceps Femoris	Ischial Tuberosity, Linea Aspera	Head of Fibula, Lateral Condyle of Tibia	Sciatic-Tibial portion and Common Peroneal Portion
Semimembranosus	Ischial Tuberosity	Upper Medial Tibia	Sciatic-Tibial Portion
Semitendinosus	Ischial Tuberosity	Upper Medial Tibia	Sciatic-Tibial Portion

Musculature/Innervation Review of the Calf and Foot

Muscle	Origin	Insertion	Nerve
Tibialis Anterior	Upper 2/3 Lateral Tibia and Interosseous Membrane	1st Cuneiform and Base of 1st Metatarsal	Deep Peroneal
Extensor Digitorum Longus	Upper 2/3 Fibula and Interosseous Membrane	4 Tendons-Distal Middle Phalanges	Deep Peroneal
Extensor Hallucis Longus	Middle 1/3 of Anterior Fibula	Base of Distal Phalanx of Big Toe	Deep Peroneal
Peroneus Tertius	Distal Fibula	Base of 5th Metatarsal	Deep Peroneal
Extensor Hallucis Brevis	Dorsal Calcaneus	Extensor Digitorum Longus Tendons	Deep Peroneal
Peroneus Longus	Upper 2/3 Lateral Fibula	1st Metatarsal and 1st Cuneiform	Superficial Peroneal
Peroneus Brevis	Lateral Distal Fibula	5th Metatarsal Tuberosity	Superficial Peroneal
Soleus	Upper Shaft of Fibula	Calcaneus via Achilles Tendon	Tibial
Flexor Digitorum Longus	Middle 1/3 of Posterior Tibia	Base of Distal Phalanx of Lateral 4 Toes	Tibial
Flexor Hallucis Longus	Middle and Lower 1/3 of Posterior Tibia	Distal Phalanx of Big Toe	Tibial
Tibialis Posterior	Posterior Upper Tibia, Fibula	Navicular Bone and 1st Cuneiform	Tibial
Popliteus	Upper Posterior Tibia	Lateral Condyle of Femur	Tibial
Flexor Digitorum Brevis	Calcaneus	Middle Phalanges of Lateral 4 Toes	Medial Plantar
Abductor Hallucis	Calcaneus	Medial Proximal Phalanx of Big Toe	Medial Plantar
Abductor Digiti Brevis	Calcaneus	Lateral Proximal Phalanx of Big Toe	Lateral Plantar
Quadratus Plantae	Lateral and Medial Side of the Calcaneus	Tendons of Flexor Digitorum Longus	Lateral Plantar
Lumbricals	Tendons of Flexor Digitorum Longus	Extensor Tendons of Toes	Medial Plantar/Lateral Plantar
Flexor Hallucis Brevis	Cuboid Bone	Splits on Base of Proximal Phalanx of Big Toe	Medial Plantar
Flexor Digiti Minimi Brevis	Base of 5th Metatarsal	Base of Proximal Phalanx of Little Toe	Lateral Plantar

Abductor Hallucis	Metatarsals 2-4	Base of Proximal Phalanx of Big Toe	Lateral Plantar
Interossei	Sides of Metatarsal Bones	Base of 1st Phalanx and Extensor Tendons	Lateral Plantar

CPR Guidelines for Professional Rescuers

Topic	Adult	Child	Infant
	Past puberty	1 y/o - puberty	Under 1 y/o
Conscious Choking	abdominal thrusts (or chest thrusts in pregnant/obese)	abdominal thrusts	5 back slaps and 5 chest thrusts in infant
Unconscious Choking	Begin chest compression. Look in the victim's mouth for foreign body before giving breaths.		
Rescue Breaths Normal breath given over 1 second until chest rises.	10-12 breaths per minute (1 breath every 6-8 seconds)	12-20 breaths per minute (1 breath every 3-5 seconds)	20 breaths per minute (1 breath every 3 seconds)
Chest Compressions to Ventilation Ratios (Single Rescuer)	30:2		
Chest Compressions to Ventilation Ratios (Two Rescuer)	30:2	15:2	
Chest Compression rate	At least 100/minute		
Chest Compression Land Marking Method	two hands center of the chest, even with nipples	one hand center of the chest even with nipples	2 or 3 fingers, just below the nipple line at the center of the chest
Chest Compression Depth	At least 2" compression (hands overlapping)	about 2" compression or 1/3 the AP diameter (only heel of one hand)	about 1 ½" compression or 1/3 the AP diameter (2 fingers)
Activate Emergency Response System	As soon as you realize that the victim is unresponsive	After 5 cycles of CPR	After 5 cycles of CPR

Checklist:

- Check the scene
- Check for responsiveness – ask, "Are you OK?"
- Adult - call 911, then administer CPR
- Child/Infant – administer CPR for 5 cycles, then call 911
- Open victim's airway and check for breathing
- Two rescue breaths should be given, 1 second each, and should produce a visible chest rise
- If the air does not go in, reposition and try 2 breaths again
- Check victim's pulse – chest compressions are recommended if an infant or child has a rate less than 60 per minute with signs of poor perfusion
- Continue 30:2 ratio until victim moves, AED is brought to the scene, or professional help arrives

Special Report: Pharmacology Generic/Trade Names of 50+ Key Drugs in Medicine

Brand Name	Generic
Synthroid	Levothyroxine
Crestor	Rosuvastatin
Ventolin	Albuterol
Nexium	Esomeprazole
Advair	Fluticasone / Salmeterol
Lantus	Insulin glargine
Vyvanse	Lisdexamfetamine
Lyrica	Pregabalin
Spiriva	Tiotropium
Januvia	Sitagliptin
Abilify	Aripiprazole
Symbicort	Budesonide / Formoterol
Tamiflu	Oseltamivir
Cialis	Tadalafil
Viagra	Sildenafil
Suboxone	Buprenorphine
Zetia	Ezetimibe
Xarelto	Rivaroxaban
Bystolic	Nebivolol
Celebrex	Celecoxib
Nasonex	Mometasone furoate
Namenda	Memantine
Flovent	Fluticasone
Oxycontin	Oxycodone
Diovan	Valsartan
Voltaren	Diclofenac
Dexilant	Dexlansoprazole
Benicar	Olmesartan
Vesicare	Solifenacin
Lumigan	Bimatoprost
Pataday	Olopatadine
Travatan	Travoprost
Toprol-XL	Metoprolol
Pristiq	Desvenlafaxine
Invokana	Canagliflozin
Strattera	Atomoxetine
Seroquel	Quetiapine
Focalin	Dexmethylphenidate
Victoza	Liraglutide
Exelon	Rivastigmine
Tradjenta	Linagliptin
Enbrel	Etanercept
Onglyza	Saxagliptin
Ranexa	Ranolazine

Truvada	Emtricitabine / Tenofovir
Welchol	Colesevelam
Linzess	Linaclotide
Latuda	Lurasidone
Alphagan	Brimonidine
Viibryd	Vilazodone
Effient	Prasugrel
Norvir	Ritonavir
Amitiza	Lubiprostone
Uloric	Febuxostat
Lotemax	Loteprednol

Special Report: Difficult Patients

Every professional will eventually get a difficult patient on their list of responsibilities. These patients can be mentally, physically, and emotionally combative in many different environments. Consequently, care of these patients should be conducted in a manner for personal and self-protection of the professional. Some of the key guidelines are as follows:

1. Never allow yourself to be cornered in a room with the patient positioned between you and the door.
2. Don't escalate the tension with verbal bantering. Basically, don't argue with the patient or resident.
3. Ask permission before performing any normal tasks in a patient's room whenever possible.
4. Discuss your concerns with nursing staff. Consult the floor supervisor if necessary, especially when safety is an issue.
5. Get help from other support staff when offering care. Get a witness if you are anticipating abuse of any kind.
6. Remove yourself from the situation if you are concerned about your personal safety at all times.
7. If attacked, defend yourself with the force necessary for self-protection and attempt to separate from the patient.
8. Be aware of the patient's medical and mental history prior to entering the patient's room.
9. Don't put yourself in a position to be hurt.
10. Get the necessary help for all transfers, bathing and dressing activities from other staff members for difficult patients.
11. Respect the resident and patient's personal property.
12. Get assistance quickly, via the call bell or vocal projection, if a situation becomes violent or abuse.
13. Immediately seek medical treatment if injured.
14. Fill out an incident report for proper documentation of the occurrence.
15. Protect other patients from abusive behavior.

Special Report: Guidelines for Standard Precautions

Standard precautions are precautions taken to avoid contracting various diseases and preventing the spread of disease to those who have compromised immunity. Some of these diseases include human immunodeficiency virus (HIV), acquired immunodeficiency syndrome (AIDS), and hepatitis B (HBV). Standard precautions are needed since many diseases do not display signs or symptoms in their early stages. Standard precautions mean to treat all body fluids/substances as if they were contaminated. These body fluids include but are not limited to the following blood, semen, vaginal secretions, breast milk, amniotic fluid, feces, urine, peritoneal fluid, synovial fluid, cerebrospinal fluid, secretions from the nasal and oral cavities, and lacrimal and sweat gland excretions. This means that standard precautions should be used with all patients.

1. A shield for the eyes and face must be used if there is a possibility of splashes from blood and body fluids.
2. If possibility of blood or body fluids being splashed on clothing, you must wear a plastic apron.
3. Gloves must be worn if you could possibly come in contact with blood or body fluids. They are also needed if you are going to touch something that may have come in contact with blood or body fluids.
4. Hands must be washed even if you were wearing gloves. Hands must be washed and gloves must be changed between patients. Wash hands with at a dime size amount of soap and warm water for about 30 seconds. Singing "Mary had a little lamb" is approximately 30 seconds.
5. Blood and body fluid spills must be cleansed and disinfected using a solution of one part bleach to 10 parts water or your hospitals accepted method.
6. Used needles must be separated from clean needles. Throw both the needle and the syringe away in the sharps' container. The sharps' container is mad of puncture proof material.
7. Take extra care in performing high-risk activities that include puncturing the skin and cutting the skin.
8. CPR equipment to be used in a hospital must include resuscitation bags and mouthpieces.

Special precautions must be taken to dispose of biomedical waste. Biomedical waste includes but is not limited to the following laboratory waste, pathology waste, liquid waste from suction, all sharp object, bladder catheters, chest tubes, IV tubes, and drainage containers. Biomedical waste is removed from a facility by trained biomedical waste disposers.

The health care professional is legally and ethically responsible for adhering to standard precautions. They may prevent you from contracting a fatal disease or from a patient contracting a disease from you that could be deadly.

Special Report: Basic Review of Types of Fractures

A fracture is defined as a break in a bone that may sometimes involve cartilaginous structures. A fracture can be classified according to its cause or the type of break. The following definitions are used to describe breaks.

1. Traumatic fracture – break in a bone resulting from injury
2. Spontaneous fracture – break in a bone resulting from disease
3. Pathologic fracture – another name for a spontaneous fracture
4. Compound fracture – occurs when fracture bone is exposed to the outside by an opening in the skin
5. Simple fracture - occurs when a break is contained within the skin
6. Greenstick fracture - a traumatic break that is incomplete and occurs on the convex surface of the bend in the bone
7. Fissured fracture – a traumatic break that involves an incomplete longitudinal break
8. Comminuted fracture – a traumatic break that involves a complete fracture that results in several bony fragments
9. Transverse fracture – a traumatic break that is complete and occurs at a right angle to the axis of the bone
10. Oblique fracture- a traumatic break that occurs at an angle other than a right angle to the axis of the bone.
11. Spiral fracture – a traumatic break that occurs by twisting a bone with extreme force

A compound fracture is much more dangerous than a simple break. This is due to the break in skin that can allow microorganisms to infect the injured tissue. When a fracture occurs, blood vessels within the bone and its periosteum are disrupted. The periosteum, covering of fibrous connective tissue on the surface of the bone, may also be damaged or torn.

How to Overcome Test Anxiety

Just the thought of taking a test is enough to make most people a little nervous. A test is an important event that can have a long-term impact on your future, so it's important to take it seriously and it's natural to feel anxious about performing well. But just because anxiety is normal, that doesn't mean that it's helpful in test taking, or that you should simply accept it as part of your life. Anxiety can have a variety of effects. These effects can be mild, like making you feel slightly nervous, or severe, like blocking your ability to focus or remember even a simple detail.

If you experience test anxiety—whether severe or mild—it's important to know how to beat it. To discover this, first you need to understand what causes test anxiety.

Causes of Test Anxiety

While we often think of anxiety as an uncontrollable emotional state, it can actually be caused by simple, practical things. One of the most common causes of test anxiety is that a person does not feel adequately prepared for their test. This feeling can be the result of many different issues such as poor study habits or lack of organization, but the most common culprit is time management. Starting to study too late, failing to organize your study time to cover all of the material, or being distracted while you study will mean that you're not well prepared for the test. This may lead to cramming the night before, which will cause you to be physically and mentally exhausted for the test. Poor time management also contributes to feelings of stress, fear, and hopelessness as you realize you are not well prepared but don't know what to do about it.

Other times, test anxiety is not related to your preparation for the test but comes from unresolved fear. This may be a past failure on a test, or poor performance on tests in general. It may come from comparing yourself to others who seem to be performing better or from the stress of living up to expectations. Anxiety may be driven by fears of the future—how failure on this test would affect your educational and career goals. These fears are often completely irrational, but they can still negatively impact your test performance.

> **Review Video:** <u>3 Reasons You Have Test Anxiety</u>
> Visit mometrix.com/academy and enter code: 428468

Elements of Test Anxiety

As mentioned earlier, test anxiety is considered to be an emotional state, but it has physical and mental components as well. Sometimes you may not even realize that you are suffering from test anxiety until you notice the physical symptoms. These can include trembling hands, rapid heartbeat, sweating, nausea, and tense muscles. Extreme anxiety may lead to fainting or vomiting. Obviously, any of these symptoms can have a negative impact on testing. It is important to recognize them as soon as they begin to occur so that you can address the problem before it damages your performance.

> **Review Video: 3 Ways to Tell You Have Test Anxiety**
> Visit mometrix.com/academy and enter code: 927847

The mental components of test anxiety include trouble focusing and inability to remember learned information. During a test, your mind is on high alert, which can help you recall information and stay focused for an extended period of time. However, anxiety interferes with your mind's natural processes, causing you to blank out, even on the questions you know well. The strain of testing during anxiety makes it difficult to stay focused, especially on a test that may take several hours. Extreme anxiety can take a huge mental toll, making it difficult not only to recall test information but even to understand the test questions or pull your thoughts together.

> **Review Video: How Test Anxiety Affects Memory**
> Visit mometrix.com/academy and enter code: 609003

Effects of Test Anxiety

Test anxiety is like a disease—if left untreated, it will get progressively worse. Anxiety leads to poor performance, and this reinforces the feelings of fear and failure, which in turn lead to poor performances on subsequent tests. It can grow from a mild nervousness to a crippling condition. If allowed to progress, test anxiety can have a big impact on your schooling, and consequently on your future.

Test anxiety can spread to other parts of your life. Anxiety on tests can become anxiety in any stressful situation, and blanking on a test can turn into panicking in a job situation. But fortunately, you don't have to let anxiety rule your testing and determine your grades. There are a number of relatively simple steps you can take to move past anxiety and function normally on a test and in the rest of life.

> **Review Video: How Test Anxiety Impacts Your Grades**
> Visit mometrix.com/academy and enter code: 939819

Physical Steps for Beating Test Anxiety

While test anxiety is a serious problem, the good news is that it can be overcome. It doesn't have to control your ability to think and remember information. While it may take time, you can begin taking steps today to beat anxiety.

Just as your first hint that you may be struggling with anxiety comes from the physical symptoms, the first step to treating it is also physical. Rest is crucial for having a clear, strong mind. If you are tired, it is much easier to give in to anxiety. But if you establish good sleep habits, your body and mind will be ready to perform optimally, without the strain of exhaustion. Additionally, sleeping well helps you to retain information better, so you're more likely to recall the answers when you see the test questions.

Getting good sleep means more than going to bed on time. It's important to allow your brain time to relax. Take study breaks from time to time so it doesn't get overworked, and don't study right before bed. Take time to rest your mind before trying to rest your body, or you may find it difficult to fall asleep.

> **Review Video: The Importance of Sleep for Your Brain**
> Visit mometrix.com/academy and enter code: 319338

Along with sleep, other aspects of physical health are important in preparing for a test. Good nutrition is vital for good brain function. Sugary foods and drinks may give a burst of energy but this burst is followed by a crash, both physically and emotionally. Instead, fuel your body with protein and vitamin-rich foods.

Also, drink plenty of water. Dehydration can lead to headaches and exhaustion, especially if your brain is already under stress from the rigors of the test. Particularly if your test is a long one, drink water during the breaks. And if possible, take an energy-boosting snack to eat between sections.

> **Review Video: How Diet Can Affect your Mood**
> Visit mometrix.com/academy and enter code: 624317

Along with sleep and diet, a third important part of physical health is exercise. Maintaining a steady workout schedule is helpful, but even taking 5-minute study breaks to walk can help get your blood pumping faster and clear your head. Exercise also releases endorphins, which contribute to a positive feeling and can help combat test anxiety.

When you nurture your physical health, you are also contributing to your mental health. If your body is healthy, your mind is much more likely to be healthy as well. So take time to rest, nourish your body with healthy food and water, and get moving as much as possible. Taking these physical steps will make you stronger and more able to take the mental steps necessary to overcome test anxiety.

> **Review Video: How to Stay Healthy and Prevent Test Anxiety**
> Visit mometrix.com/academy and enter code: 877894

Mental Steps for Beating Test Anxiety

Working on the mental side of test anxiety can be more challenging, but as with the physical side, there are clear steps you can take to overcome it. As mentioned earlier, test anxiety often stems from lack of preparation, so the obvious solution is to prepare for the test. Effective studying may be the most important weapon you have for beating test anxiety, but you can and should employ several other mental tools to combat fear.

First, boost your confidence by reminding yourself of past success—tests or projects that you aced. If you're putting as much effort into preparing for this test as you did for those, there's no reason you should expect to fail here. Work hard to prepare; then trust your preparation.

Second, surround yourself with encouraging people. It can be helpful to find a study group, but be sure that the people you're around will encourage a positive attitude. If you spend time with others who are anxious or cynical, this will only contribute to your own anxiety. Look for others who are motivated to study hard from a desire to succeed, not from a fear of failure.

Third, reward yourself. A test is physically and mentally tiring, even without anxiety, and it can be helpful to have something to look forward to. Plan an activity following the test, regardless of the outcome, such as going to a movie or getting ice cream.

When you are taking the test, if you find yourself beginning to feel anxious, remind yourself that you know the material. Visualize successfully completing the test. Then take a few deep, relaxing breaths and return to it. Work through the questions carefully but with confidence, knowing that you are capable of succeeding.

Developing a healthy mental approach to test taking will also aid in other areas of life. Test anxiety affects more than just the actual test—it can be damaging to your mental health and even contribute to depression. It's important to beat test anxiety before it becomes a problem for more than testing.

> **Review Video: Test Anxiety and Depression**
> Visit mometrix.com/academy and enter code: 904704

Study Strategy

Being prepared for the test is necessary to combat anxiety, but what does being prepared look like? You may study for hours on end and still not feel prepared. What you need is a strategy for test prep. The next few pages outline our recommended steps to help you plan out and conquer the challenge of preparation.

Step 1: Scope Out the Test

Learn everything you can about the format (multiple choice, essay, etc.) and what will be on the test. Gather any study materials, course outlines, or sample exams that may be available. Not only will this help you to prepare, but knowing what to expect can help to alleviate test anxiety.

Step 2: Map Out the Material

Look through the textbook or study guide and make note of how many chapters or sections it has. Then divide these over the time you have. For example, if a book has 15 chapters and you have five days to study, you need to cover three chapters each day. Even better, if you have the time, leave an extra day at the end for overall review after you have gone through the material in depth.

If time is limited, you may need to prioritize the material. Look through it and make note of which sections you think you already have a good grasp on, and which need review. While you are studying, skim quickly through the familiar sections and take more time on the challenging parts. Write out your plan so you don't get lost as you go. Having a written plan also helps you feel more in control of the study, so anxiety is less likely to arise from feeling overwhelmed at the amount to cover. A sample plan may look like this:

- Day 1: Skim chapters 1–4, study chapter 5 (especially pages 31–33)
- Day 2: Study chapters 6–7, skim chapters 8–9
- Day 3: Skim chapter 10, study chapters 11–12 (especially pages 87–90)
- Day 4: Study chapters 13–15
- Day 5: Overall review (focus most on chapters 5, 6, and 12), take practice test

Step 3: Gather Your Tools

Decide what study method works best for you. Do you prefer to highlight in the book as you study and then go back over the highlighted portions? Or do you type out notes of the important information? Or is it helpful to make flashcards that you can carry with you? Assemble the pens, index cards, highlighters, post-it notes, and any other materials you may need so you won't be distracted by getting up to find things while you study.

If you're having a hard time retaining the information or organizing your notes, experiment with different methods. For example, try color-coding by subject with colored pens, highlighters, or post-it notes. If you learn better by hearing, try recording yourself reading your notes so you can listen while in the car, working out, or simply sitting at your desk. Ask a friend to quiz you from your flashcards, or try teaching someone the material to solidify it in your mind.

Step 4: Create Your Environment

It's important to avoid distractions while you study. This includes both the obvious distractions like visitors and the subtle distractions like an uncomfortable chair (or a too-comfortable couch that makes you want to fall asleep). Set up the best study environment possible: good lighting and a comfortable work area. If background music helps you focus, you may want to turn it on, but otherwise keep the room quiet. If you are using a computer to take notes, be sure you don't have any other windows open, especially applications like social media, games, or anything else that could distract you. Silence your phone and turn off notifications. Be sure to keep water close by so you stay hydrated while you study (but avoid unhealthy drinks and snacks).

Also, take into account the best time of day to study. Are you freshest first thing in the morning? Try to set aside some time then to work through the material. Is your mind clearer in the afternoon or evening? Schedule your study session then. Another method is to study at the same time of day that you will take the test, so that your brain gets used to working on the material at that time and will be ready to focus at test time.

Step 5: Study!

Once you have done all the study preparation, it's time to settle into the actual studying. Sit down, take a few moments to settle your mind so you can focus, and begin to follow your study plan. Don't give in to distractions or let yourself procrastinate. This is your time to prepare so you'll be ready to fearlessly approach the test. Make the most of the time and stay focused.

Of course, you don't want to burn out. If you study too long you may find that you're not retaining the information very well. Take regular study breaks. For example, taking five minutes out of every hour to walk briskly, breathing deeply and swinging your arms, can help your mind stay fresh.

As you get to the end of each chapter or section, it's a good idea to do a quick review. Remind yourself of what you learned and work on any difficult parts. When you feel that you've mastered the material, move on to the next part. At the end of your study session, briefly skim through your notes again.

But while review is helpful, cramming last minute is NOT. If at all possible, work ahead so that you won't need to fit all your study into the last day. Cramming overloads your brain with more information than it can process and retain, and your tired mind may struggle to recall even previously learned information when it is overwhelmed with last-minute study. Also, the urgent nature of cramming and the stress placed on your brain contribute to anxiety. You'll be more likely to go to the test feeling unprepared and having trouble thinking clearly.

So don't cram, and don't stay up late before the test, even just to review your notes at a leisurely pace. Your brain needs rest more than it needs to go over the information again. In fact, plan to finish your studies by noon or early afternoon the day before the test. Give your brain the rest of the day to relax or focus on other things, and get a good night's sleep. Then you will be fresh for the test and better able to recall what you've studied.

Step 6: Take a practice test

Many courses offer sample tests, either online or in the study materials. This is an excellent resource to check whether you have mastered the material, as well as to prepare for the test format and environment.

Check the test format ahead of time: the number of questions, the type (multiple choice, free response, etc.), and the time limit. Then create a plan for working through them. For example, if you have 30 minutes to take a 60-question test, your limit is 30 seconds per question. Spend less time on the questions you know well so that you can take more time on the difficult ones.

If you have time to take several practice tests, take the first one open book, with no time limit. Work through the questions at your own pace and make sure you fully understand them. Gradually work up to taking a test under test conditions: sit at a desk with all study materials put away and set a timer. Pace yourself to make sure you finish the test with time to spare and go back to check your answers if you have time.

After each test, check your answers. On the questions you missed, be sure you understand why you missed them. Did you misread the question (tests can use tricky wording)? Did you forget the information? Or was it something you hadn't learned? Go back and study any shaky areas that the practice tests reveal.

Taking these tests not only helps with your grade, but also aids in combating test anxiety. If you're already used to the test conditions, you're less likely to worry about it, and working through tests until you're scoring well gives you a confidence boost. Go through the practice tests until you feel comfortable, and then you can go into the test knowing that you're ready for it.

Test Tips

On test day, you should be confident, knowing that you've prepared well and are ready to answer the questions. But aside from preparation, there are several test day strategies you can employ to maximize your performance.

First, as stated before, get a good night's sleep the night before the test (and for several nights before that, if possible). Go into the test with a fresh, alert mind rather than staying up late to study.

Try not to change too much about your normal routine on the day of the test. It's important to eat a nutritious breakfast, but if you normally don't eat breakfast at all, consider eating just a protein bar. If you're a coffee drinker, go ahead and have your normal coffee. Just make sure you time it so that the caffeine doesn't wear off right in the middle of your test. Avoid sugary beverages, and drink enough water to stay hydrated but not so much that you need a restroom break 10 minutes into the test. If your test isn't first thing in the morning, consider going for a walk or doing a light workout before the test to get your blood flowing.

Allow yourself enough time to get ready, and leave for the test with plenty of time to spare so you won't have the anxiety of scrambling to arrive in time. Another reason to be early is to select a good seat. It's helpful to sit away from doors and windows, which can be distracting. Find a good seat, get out your supplies, and settle your mind before the test begins.

When the test begins, start by going over the instructions carefully, even if you already know what to expect. Make sure you avoid any careless mistakes by following the directions.

Then begin working through the questions, pacing yourself as you've practiced. If you're not sure on an answer, don't spend too much time on it, and don't let it shake your confidence. Either skip it and come back later, or eliminate as many wrong answers as possible and guess among the remaining ones. Don't dwell on these questions as you continue—put them out of your mind and focus on what lies ahead.

Be sure to read all of the answer choices, even if you're sure the first one is the right answer. Sometimes you'll find a better one if you keep reading. But don't second-guess yourself if you do immediately know the answer. Your gut instinct is usually right. Don't let test anxiety rob you of the information you know.

If you have time at the end of the test (and if the test format allows), go back and review your answers. Be cautious about changing any, since your first instinct tends to be correct, but make sure you didn't misread any of the questions or accidentally mark the wrong answer choice. Look over any you skipped and make an educated guess.

At the end, leave the test feeling confident. You've done your best, so don't waste time worrying about your performance or wishing you could change anything. Instead, celebrate the successful completion of this test. And finally, use this test to learn how to deal with anxiety even better next time.

Review Video: 5 Tips to Beat Test Anxiety
Visit mometrix.com/academy and enter code: 570656

Important Qualification

Not all anxiety is created equal. If your test anxiety is causing major issues in your life beyond the classroom or testing center, or if you are experiencing troubling physical symptoms related to your anxiety, it may be a sign of a serious physiological or psychological condition. If this sounds like your situation, we strongly encourage you to seek professional help.

Thank You

We at Mometrix would like to extend our heartfelt thanks to you, our friend and patron, for allowing us to play a part in your journey. It is a privilege to serve people from all walks of life who are unified in their commitment to building the best future they can for themselves.

The preparation you devote to these important testing milestones may be the most valuable educational opportunity you have for making a real difference in your life. We encourage you to put your heart into it—that feeling of succeeding, overcoming, and yes, conquering will be well worth the hours you've invested.

We want to hear your story, your struggles and your successes, and if you see any opportunities for us to improve our materials so we can help others even more effectively in the future, please share that with us as well. **The team at Mometrix would be absolutely thrilled to hear from you!** So please, send us an email (support@mometrix.com) and let's stay in touch.

If you'd like some additional help, check out these other resources we offer for your exam:

http://MometrixFlashcards.com/PSB

Additional Bonus Material

Due to our efforts to try to keep this book to a manageable length, we've created a link that will give you access to all of your additional bonus material.

Please visit https://www.mometrix.com/bonus948/psbpn to access the information.

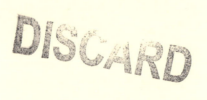